FIRST AID
FOR
CHILDREN
FAST

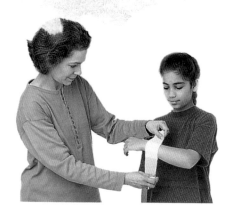

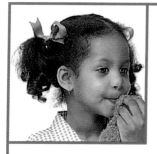

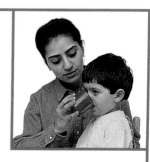

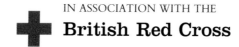

IN ASSOCIATION WITH THE
British Red Cross

FIRST AID
FOR
CHILDREN
FAST

Chief Medical Advisor: British Red Cross
Dr Gordon Paterson

A Dorling Kindersley Book

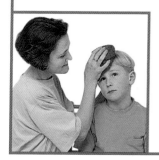

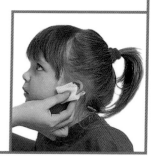

LONDON, NEW YORK, MUNICH, MELBOURNE, DELHI

BRITISH RED CROSS
Chief Medical Advisor Dr J Gordon Paterson FFPHM FRCPE DRCOG DCM
Project Manager Dr Vivien J Armstrong FRCA DRCOG PGCE

DORLING KINDERSLEY LIMITED
Editor Joanna Benwell
Senior Editor Janet Mohun

Art Editors Sara Freeman, Floyd Sayers
DTP Designer Julian Dams

Senior Managing Editor Jemima Dunne
Managing Art Editor Louise Dick

Production Wendy Penn
Photography Gary Ombler

First published in Great Britain in 1994; revised in 1999

Second revision published 2002 by Dorling Kindersley Limited,
80 Strand, London WC2R 0RL
A Penguin Company

2 4 6 8 10 9 7 5 3 1

Copyright © 1994, 1999, 2002 Dorling Kindersley Limited, London

A CIP catalogue record for this book is available from the British Library

ISBN 0 7513 4396 X

Reproduced in Italy by GRB Editrice, Verona
Printed and bound in Italy by Graphicom

See our complete catalogue at
www.dk.com

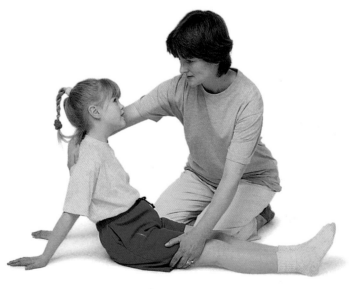

FOREWORD

I am pleased to support this British Red Cross manual – *First Aid for Children Fast*. This revision of the existing manual has been produced to bring families and carers up to date with advances in first aid that, like all aspects of medicine, constantly change in response to new clinical evidence and new technology. Updates are therefore important to maintain your skills and knowledge in line with new evidence.

Children are naturally adventurous and have enormous energy. It is not surprising, therefore, that in life's learning journey they have the potential for injuring themselves. Fortunately, they are also resilient and have the ability to recover quickly, but sometimes they need help. It is therefore very important for a child's carer to have skills in first aid.

I trust that this book will add to your skills in a practical way and that, together with your natural instincts to care for your children, it will contribute to their quick recovery from injury and illness.

Dr Gordon Paterson

Chief Medical Advisor to the British Red Cross

CONTENTS

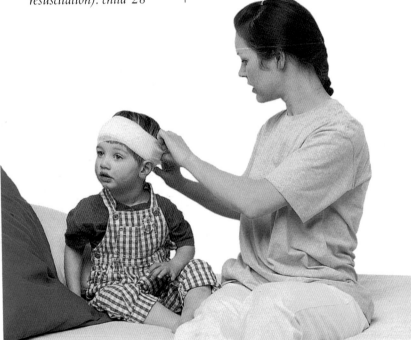

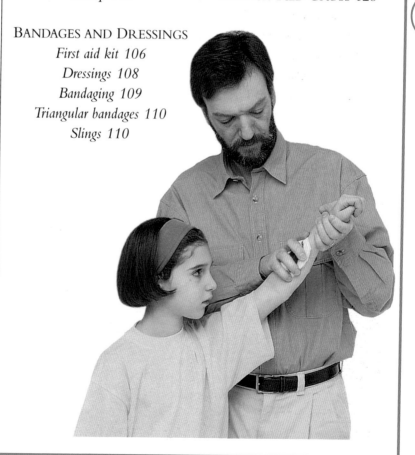

INTRODUCTION

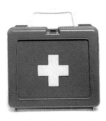

This book has been compiled primarily for parents but also for others – grandparents, teachers, childminders, babysitters, playgroup leaders – who may regularly, or even occasionally, find themselves in charge of infants and children. The content has been set out in a clear and logical way and the information presented largely in pictorial form using simple words and captions to make it very easy to follow and to understand. The first aid methods and techniques described reflect the relevant guidance set out by the Paediatric Life Support Group of the European Resuscitation Council and are current at the time of publication.

Emergencies are, by their very nature, unexpected events and require a prompt and proper response. If you follow the advice and guidance given in this book you will undoubtedly be able to give early and effective help whenever it is needed. You should be aware, however, that first aid is essentially a practical skill and your confidence and effectiveness will be greatly enhanced by expert training in a practical setting. The British Red Cross regularly runs a wide variety of first aid learning programmes, some exclusively concerned with first aid for infants and children. You can find out more about these by ringing your local British Red Cross office – the number will be in your phone book – who will be very pleased to hear from you.

Giving first aid – coping with the emergency and doing the right thing early and effectively – can be straightforward, but it can also be stressful, sometimes distasteful (especially if the child is not your own), and even dangerous. It is important that you remain in control of your feelings and avoid any tendency to rash action that could result in additional harm to an injured child or to yourself. You cannot give effective help if you yourself become a casualty so you must always take a little time to think before you act. This book is intended to help you to do the right thing at the right time – safely and effectively.

How to use this book

This book covers first aid treatment for everything from minor cuts and grazes to resuscitation. For every condition a series of photographs shows you exactly what to do in an emergency. Key pieces of information are indicated on the photographs and supplementary advice can be found alongside in the step-by-step text.

The injuries are organised by type, in sections such as WOUNDS AND BLEEDING and BITES AND STINGS. However, in an emergency, the thumbnail index on the back cover will direct you straight to the relevant page.

There are also sections, such as ACTION IN AN EMERGENCY and BANDAGES AND DRESSINGS, that contain information for general reference.

Key signs and symptoms help you to recognise the conditions

Clear photographs illustrate every step of treatment

Annotations highlight essential action

The quick reference index on the back cover gives instant access to major first aid emergencies

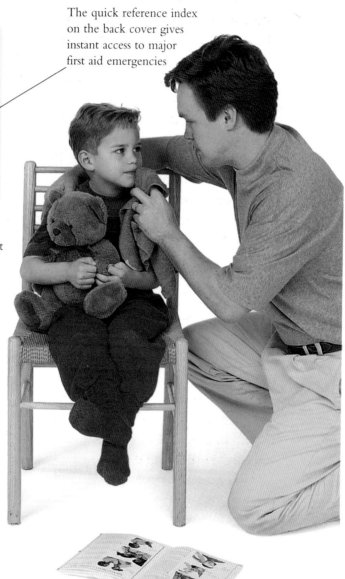

Symbols highlight the action necessary for further medical attention

Cross-references direct you to other pages where information is given about associated injuries

Guide to the symbols
The following symbols and instructions appear if your child needs further medical attention:

C CALL A DOCTOR
(Telephone for further advice.)

✚ TAKE YOUR CHILD TO HOSPITAL
(Your child needs to be seen in the Accident and Emergency department.)

☎ CALL AN AMBULANCE
(Your child needs urgent medical attention and is best transported by ambulance to hospital.)

ACTION IN AN EMERGENCY

**In any emergency, particularly one involving children,
it is important to keep calm and act logically. Remember four steps:**

1 Assess the situation

- What happened?
- How did it happen?
- Is there more than one injured child?
- Is there any continuing danger?
- Is there anyone who can help?
- Do I need an ambulance?

2 Think of safety

- Do not risk injuring yourself – you cannot help if you become a casualty
- Remove any source of danger from your child
- Move your child only if you must and do so very carefully

3 Treat serious injuries first

In children, there are two conditions that immediately threaten life:
- *Inability to breathe* (see ABC OF RESUSCITATION p.14)
- *Serious bleeding* – this is usually obvious and can be brought under control
  (see BLEEDING p.46)

If more than one child is injured go quickly to the quiet one – he may be unconscious.

4 Get help

Shout for help early and ask others to:
- Make the area safe
- Help with first aid
- Call a doctor or an ambulance
- Move a child to safety, if necessary

Telephoning for help

When you call the emergency services, ask for an
ambulance and give the following information:

- Your telephone number
- The location of the accident
- The type of accident
- The number, sex, and age of the casualties
- Details about their condition
- Details of any hazards such as gas, power line damage, or fog

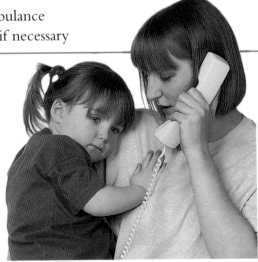

FIRE

Have an escape plan

Before an emergency happens, decide:
- *How would you get out of each room?*
- *How do you help babies and small children?*
- *Where will you meet when you've escaped?*

CHIP PAN FIRE • *Turn off stove or hob* • *Cover pan with lid, wet tea towel, or fire blanket – leave this on for half an hour* • *DO NOT throw water over the flames* • *If not under control, close the door, get everyone out of the house, call the fire brigade*

Escaping from a fire

1 Feel the door. If the door is cool, leave the room. If it is hot, see opposite.

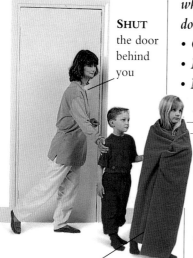

SHUT the door behind you

REMEMBER • *Carry out babies and toddlers* • *Children over six should look after only themselves when escaping – don't ask them to do anything else.*
- *Close all doors behind you*
- *Meet outside your house*
- *NEVER go back inside* • *Phone for help from somewhere else*

2 If the door is hot, don't open it. Go to the window.

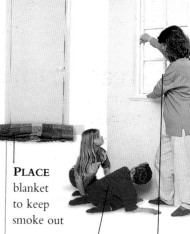

IF *you have to escape through the window, slide your child out, hang onto him, then ask him to drop to the ground. Slide out yourself, hang from the ledge, then drop. If you have to break the glass first, put a blanket over the frame before escaping.*

LEAVE quickly
DO NOT GO BACK

PLACE blanket to keep smoke out

KEEP children low, where air is clearest

OPEN window, call for help

11

Clothing on fire

If clothing is on fire:

Stop your child moving as movement will fan the flames.
Drop him to the floor to stop him burning his face and airway.
Wrap him in a coat or blanket to help smother the flames.
Roll him on the ground to put out the fire.

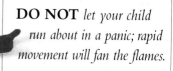

IF *water is available, lay him down, burning side uppermost, and douse him with water or a non-flammable liquid.*

DO NOT *let your child run about in a panic; rapid movement will fan the flames.*

ELECTRICAL INJURY

If an electrical current passes through a child's body, it may cause the breathing and even the heart to stop. The current may cause burns both where it enters and leaves the body. Alternating current causes muscle spasms that can prevent a child letting go of an electric cable.

> **CONTACT** *with high-voltage current, found in power lines and overhead cables, is usually fatal for a child. Severe burns result and the child may be thrown some distance from the point of contact.* **NEVER** *approach the injured child unless you are told officially that the power has been cut off, or you will be in danger from "arcing", or "jumping", high-voltage electricity.*

Low-voltage current

Children are at risk of suffering an electric shock if they play with electrical sockets or flex, or if they bring water into contact with an electrical appliance.

> **IF** *your child seems unharmed, make him rest and observe his condition.* © CALL A DOCTOR

1 Break the contact by switching off the current at the mains.

2 If you cannot switch off the current, stand on dry insulating material such as telephone books or a wooden box. Use a wooden broom handle or chair to push your child's limbs away from the source.

> **IF** *your child loses consciousness, assess his condition (see* UNCONSCIOUS BABY *p.16;* CHILD *p.22). Cool any burns with cold water (see* ELECTRICAL BURNS *p.62). Be prepared to resuscitate. If breathing, place him in the* RECOVERY POSITION.

> **DO NOT** *touch your child's skin with your hands. Pull at his clothes only as a last resort.*

STAND on insulating material

3 Without touching your child, wrap a dry towel around his feet and pull him away from the source.

PUSH the source away

☎ CALL AN AMBULANCE

WRAP a dry towel around his feet. Pull him away

DROWNING

Babies and young children can drown quickly if they slip into a pool or pond or are left unattended in a bath. Even 2.5cm (1in) of water is enough to cover a baby's nose and mouth if she falls forwards.

A CHILD may get into difficulty in open water especially if it is turbulent or very cold. Rescue him quickly. Try to reach him from the shore or bank with your hand, or with a stick. Get him dry and warm as quickly as possible (see also HYPOTHERMIA p.94).

1 Lift your child out of the water. Carry her with her head lower than her chest to reduce the risk of inhaling water.

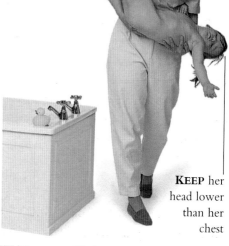

KEEP her head lower than her chest

2 **+** TAKE YOUR CHILD TO HOSPITAL, even if she seems recovered, as she may have inhaled water, causing lung damage.

The unconscious child

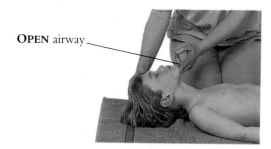

OPEN airway

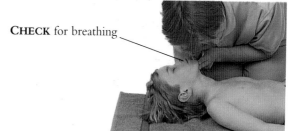

CHECK for breathing

13

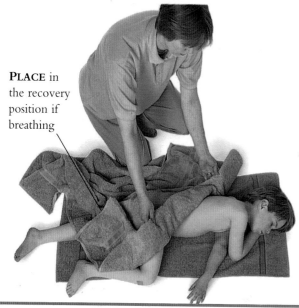

PLACE in the recovery position if breathing

Remove any wet clothing and cover him with a dry towel or blanket. Assess his condition (see UNCONSCIOUS BABY p.16; CHILD p.22). Be prepared to resuscitate. If breathing, place him in the RECOVERY POSITION.

☎ CALL AN AMBULANCE

WATER in the lungs and the effects of cold can increase resistance to rescue breathing so you may need to breathe more firmly and more slowly to get the chest to rise.

ABC OF RESUSCITATION

A baby or child who becomes unconsious may stop breathing because no oxygen reaches the brain. Lack of oxygen also slows down the heartbeat until it stops altogether. If your baby or child is unconscious and stops breathing, you need to open the airway and

breathe into the lungs (rescue breathing). If the circulation has stopped, you need to drive blood to the brain with chest compressions. This combination of rescue breathing and chest compressions is known as cardiopulmonary resuscitation (CPR).

FOR *a step-by-step guide to* RESUSCITATING A BABY *see p.16.* **FOR** *a step-by-step guide to* RESUSCITATING A CHILD *see p.22*

ASSESS your baby and act on your findings

ASSESS your child and act on your findings

TAP her shoulder

14

A is for airway

You need to open the air passage, or airway. Place one hand on the forehead and gently tilt the head back to bring the tongue away from the back of the throat. Remove any obvious obstruction from the mouth and lift the chin. If you suspect a neck injury, use the jaw thrust method to open the airway (see p.74).

For a baby

For a child

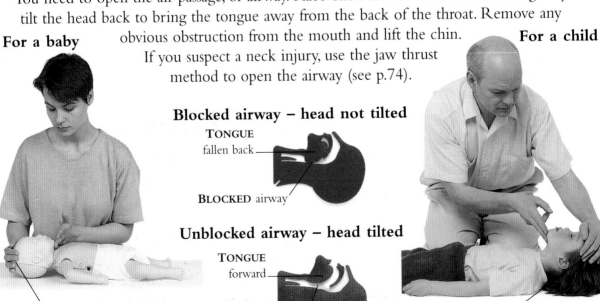

Blocked airway – head not tilted

TONGUE fallen back

BLOCKED airway

Unblocked airway – head tilted

TONGUE forward

UNBLOCKED airway

TILT the head back to clear the airway

TILT the head back to clear the airway

B is for breathing

For a baby

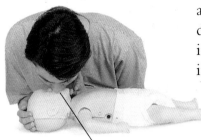

If your child is not breathing after the airway is open, take a deep breath and blow steadily into the lungs to get oxygen into the child's blood.

For a child

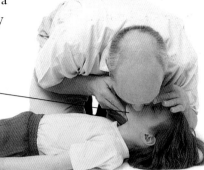

HOLD the nose and blow into the mouth

BREATHE gently into the mouth and nose until the chest rises

C is for circulation

For a baby

If your child's heart has stopped and there are no signs of circulation, giving chest compressions will drive blood through the heart and around the body. This is always combined with rescue breathing. The combination of techniques is known as cardiopulmonary resuscitation (CPR).

For a child

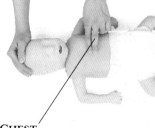

CHEST COMPRESSIONS are given with two fingers

CHEST COMPRESSIONS are given with one hand only

15

When to call an ambulance

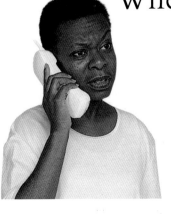

If there is somebody else present, always ask him or her to call an ambulance as soon as you realise that your child is not breathing.

If you are alone, give rescue breaths (see RESCUE BREATHING: BABY p.18; CHILD p.26) or cardiopulmonary rescuscitation (see CPR: BABY p.20; CHILD p.28), as appropriate, for about one minute before pausing to call an ambulance.

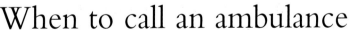

UNCONSCIOUS BABY

Assess your baby's condition

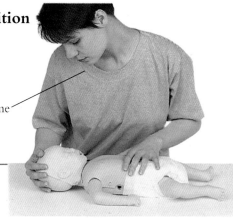

1 Check for response

- Call his name
- Tap or flick the sole of his foot

NEVER shake a baby

CALL his name

2 Shout for help

3 Open the airway

- Place one hand on the forehead and gently tilt the head back
- Remove any obvious obstruction from the mouth
- Use one finger to lift the chin

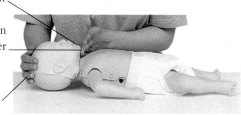

LOOK in mouth

LIFT chin with one finger

TILT head back

4 Check for breathing

- Listen for sounds of breathing
- Feel for breath on your cheek
- Look along the chest for movement
- Check for no more than ten seconds
- If breathing, go straight to step 6 (opposite)

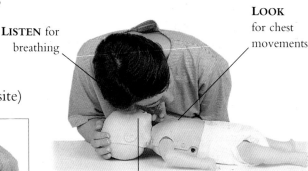

LISTEN for breathing

LOOK for chest movements

FEEL for breath on your cheek

IF NOT *breathing, give two effective rescue breaths (see p.18), then proceed to step 5 (below).*

PUT your mouth over baby's mouth and nose

5 Check for signs of circulation

- Look for breathing, coughing, and movement for no more than ten seconds

16

6 Act on your findings

Baby unconscious, breathing present

1 Treat any life-threatening injuries such as severe bleeding (p.46).

2 Cradle your baby in your arms with his head tilted down (the recovery position).

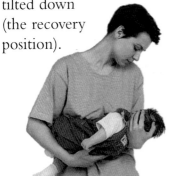

3 ☎ CALL AN AMBULANCE
Ask a helper to do this. If you have no helper, take your baby with you to the telephone.

4 Keep your baby in your arms until help arrives. Keep checking his breathing.

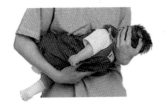

Not breathing but circulation present

1 Continue to give rescue breaths (mouth-to-mouth-and-nose) for about one minute (see overleaf).

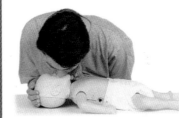

2 ☎ CALL AN AMBULANCE
Take your baby with you to the telephone, if necessary.

3 Continue giving rescue breaths until help arrives.

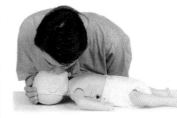

4 Check for signs of circulation every minute.

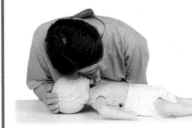

Not breathing, no signs of circulation

1 Give cardiopulmonary resuscitation (CPR) – five chest compressions followed by one rescue breath (mouth-to-mouth-and-nose) – for one minute (see p.20).

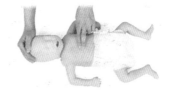

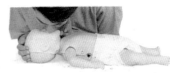

2 ☎ CALL AN AMBULANCE
Take your baby with you to the telephone, if necessary.

3 Continue giving cardiopulmonary resuscitation (CPR) until help arrives.

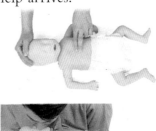

RESCUE BREATHING: BABY

To be used for an unconscious baby who is not breathing. Always attempt rescue breathing before you check for signs of circulation (see p.16).

RESUSCITATION SUMMARY

UNCONSCIOUS BABY

AIRWAY OPEN

NO BREATHING

GIVE 2 EFFECTIVE **RESCUE BREATHS**

SIGNS OF CIRCULATION PRESENT

GIVE **RESCUE BREATHS** FOR 1 MINUTE

☎ CALL AN AMBULANCE

CONTINUE GIVING **RESCUE BREATHS** UNTIL HELP ARRIVES

18

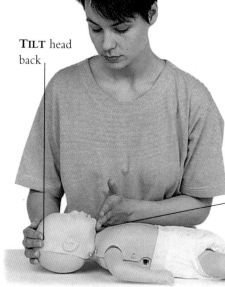

TILT head back

LIFT point of chin with one finger

1 Make sure your baby is on his back on a firm surface. Check that his airway is open. Pick out any obvious obstruction with your fingertips, but do not do a finger sweep. Lift his chin using one finger.

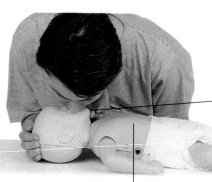

BREATHE into the baby's mouth and nose

LET the chest rise

2 Seal your lips tightly around your baby's mouth and nose. Breathe gently into the lungs until the chest rises.

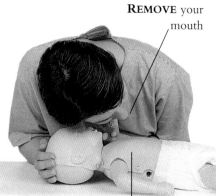

REMOVE your mouth

WATCH the chest fall back

3 Remove your mouth and let the chest fall back. A breath is effective if the chest rises and falls.

IF *your baby's chest does not rise, check his mouth again and adjust the position of his head.*

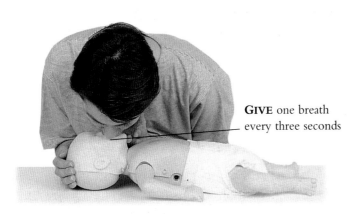

GIVE one breath
every three seconds

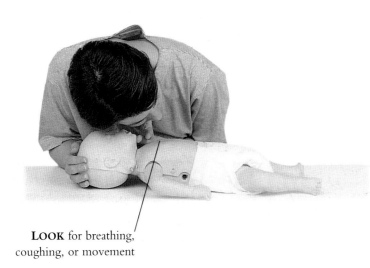

LOOK for breathing,
coughing, or movement

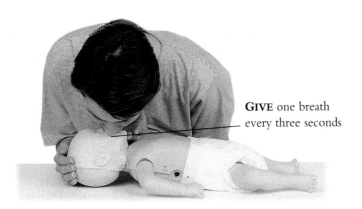

GIVE one breath
every three seconds

4 Repeat rescue breath attempts up to five times if necessary, to achieve two effective breaths.

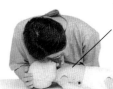

WATCH chest fall
after each breath

5 Stop and check for signs of circulation (see p.16). If these are absent, start cardiopulmonary resuscitation, or CPR, (see overleaf). Otherwise, continue to give rescue breaths for one minute, aiming for one effective breath every three seconds (about 20 breaths per minute).

6 ☎ CALL AN AMBULANCE
Take your baby with you to the telephone, if necessary.

7 Continue to give rescue breaths until help arrives. Check for signs of circulation every minute. If absent, start CPR (see overleaf).

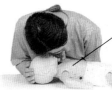

WATCH chest fall
after each breath

19

CPR (CARDIOPULMONARY RESUSCITATION) : BABY

To be used for an unconscious baby who is not breathing and has no signs of circulation (see p.16). Give CPR for a full minute before you call an ambulance.

RESUSCITATION SUMMARY

UNCONSCIOUS BABY

AIRWAY OPEN

NO BREATHING

GIVE 2 EFFECTIVE RESCUE BREATHS
(see p.18)

NO SIGNS OF CIRCULATION

CPR – 5 CHEST COMPRESSIONS, 1 RESCUE BREATH – REPEATED FOR 1 MINUTE

☎ CALL AN AMBULANCE

CONTINUE **CPR** UNTIL HELP ARRIVES

1 Place your baby on a firm surface. Place the tips of two fingers on the lower breastbone just below the nipple line.

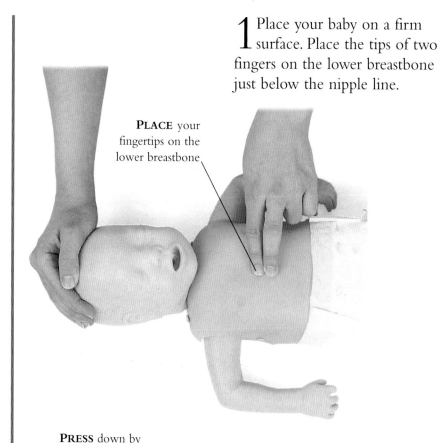

PLACE your fingertips on the lower breastbone

PRESS down by one-third of the depth of the chest

2 Press down sharply by one-third of the depth of the chest. Do this five times at a rate of 100 compressions per minute.

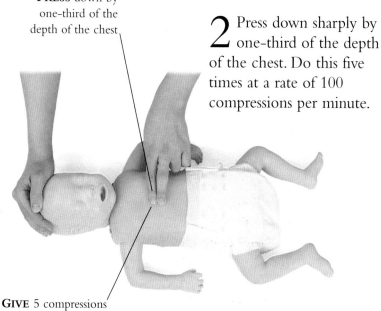

GIVE 5 compressions

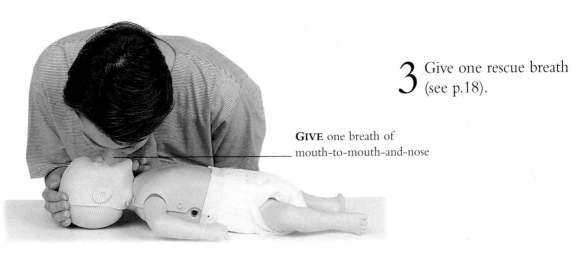

3 Give one rescue breath (see p.18).

GIVE one breath of
mouth-to-mouth-and-nose

Repeat steps 2 and 3 for about a minute

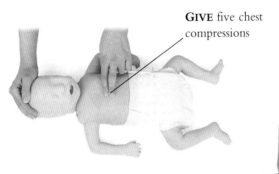

GIVE five chest
compressions

4 Continue the cycle of five chest compressions to one rescue breath for about a minute.

FOLLOW with
one breath

Repeat CPR cycles until help arrives

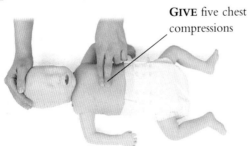

GIVE five chest
compressions

5 ☎ CALL AN AMBULANCE
If you have no helper, take your baby with you to the telephone.

6 Continue giving CPR – five chest compressions followed by one rescue breath – until the ambulance arrives.

DO NOT *stop to make circulation checks unless your baby makes a movement or takes a spontaneous breath. If breathing and circulation return, cradle your baby in your arms with his head tilted down (see p.17) and monitor him carefully until the ambulance arrives.*

FOLLOW with
one breath

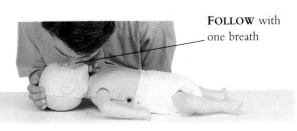

UNCONSCIOUS CHILD

Assess your child's condition

1 Check for response
- Call her name
- Tap her shoulder gently

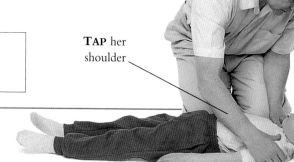

> **IF** *you suspect BACK AND NECK INJURIES, see pp. 74–75.*

TAP her
shoulder

2 Shout for help

3 Open the airway
- Place one hand on the forehead and gently tilt the head back
- Remove any obvious obstruction from the mouth.
- Use two fingers to lift the chin

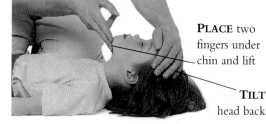

PLACE two
fingers under
chin and lift

TILT
head back

4 Check for breathing
- Listen for sounds of breathing
- Feel for breath on your cheek
- Look along the chest for movement
- Check for no more than ten seconds
- If breathing, go straight to step 6 (opposite)

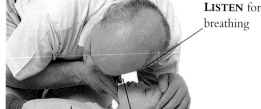

LISTEN for
breathing

> **IF NOT** *breathing, give two effective rescue breaths (see p. 26), then proceed to step 5 (below).*

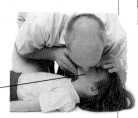

PUT your mouth over
child's mouth and breathe

LOOK for
chest movements

FEEL for
breath on
your cheek

5 Check for signs of circulation
- Look for breathing, coughing, and movement for no more than ten seconds

22

Act on your findings

Child unconscious, breathing present

1 Treat any life-threatening injuries such as severe bleeding (see p.46).

2 Place her in the recovery position (see overleaf).

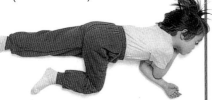

3 ☎ CALL AN AMBULANCE

4 Keep checking her breathing until help arrives and be prepared to resuscitate.

Not breathing but circulation present

1 Continue to give rescue breaths (mouth-to-mouth) for about one minute (see p.26).

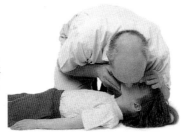

2 ☎ CALL AN AMBULANCE

3 Continue giving rescue breaths until help arrives.

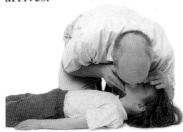

4 Check for signs of circulation every minute (after every 20 breaths).

Not breathing, no signs of circulation

1 Give cardiopulmonary resuscitation (CPR) – five chest compressions followed by one rescue breath (mouth-to-mouth) – for one minute (see p.28).

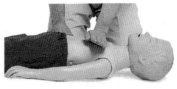

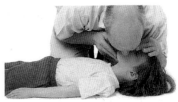

2 ☎ CALL AN AMBULANCE

3 Continue giving cardiopulmonary resuscitation (CPR) until help arrives.

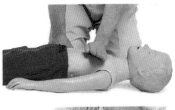

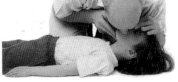

23

RECOVERY POSITION

Put your child in this position if she is unconscious, breathing and has signs of circulation (see p.22) to prevent her choking on her tongue or vomit.

BE *very careful if you think there is a broken bone. Move her so the injured side is uppermost. See BONE, JOINT AND MUSCLE INJURIES, pp.76–84.*

IF *you suspect BACK AND NECK INJURIES, see pp.74–75.*

1 Kneel beside your child. Remove spectacles and any bulky objects from her pockets. If necessary, straighten her legs. Bend the arm nearest to you so that it makes a right angle and lay it on the ground, with the palm of the hand upward.

STRAIGHTEN her legs

BEND arm nearest to you at a right angle

PLACE back of her hand on the ground

2 Bring her other arm across her chest. Hold the back of her hand against her opposite cheek.

MOVE furthest arm across her chest and bend it

PLACE back of her hand against her cheek

PLACE her foot flat on ground

CLASP under thigh of outside leg and bend at knee

3 Use your free hand to clasp gently under the thigh that is furthest from you. Carefully pull the knee up to bend the leg, leaving the foot flat on the ground.

KEEP this leg straight

SUPPORT her hand against her cheek

24

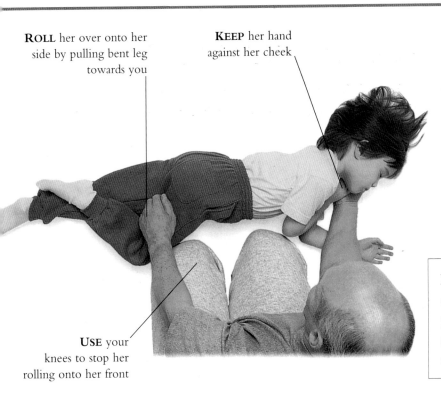

ROLL her over onto her side by pulling bent leg towards you

KEEP her hand against her cheek

USE your knees to stop her rolling onto her front

4 Keep your child's hand against her cheek to support her head. At the same time, pull on the thigh of the bent leg to roll your child towards you and onto her side.

IF *your child is already lying on her side or is on her front, you will need to adapt the steps when placing her in the recovery position.*

25

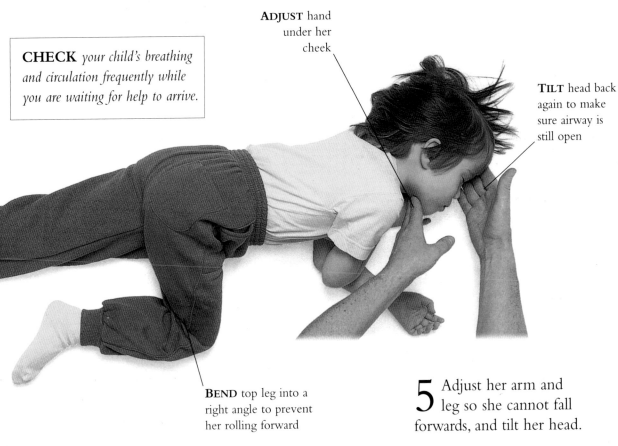

CHECK *your child's breathing and circulation frequently while you are waiting for help to arrive.*

ADJUST hand under her cheek

TILT head back again to make sure airway is still open

BEND top leg into a right angle to prevent her rolling forward

5 Adjust her arm and leg so she cannot fall forwards, and tilt her head.

☎ CALL AN AMBULANCE

RESCUE BREATHING: CHILD

**To be used for an unconscious child who is not breathing. Always attempt
rescue breathing before you check for signs of circulation (see p.22).**

**RESUSCITATION
SUMMARY**

UNCONSCIOUS CHILD

AIRWAY OPEN

NO BREATHING

GIVE 2 EFFECTIVE
RESCUE BREATHS

SIGNS OF
CIRCULATION
PRESENT

GIVE
RESCUE BREATHS
FOR 1 MINUTE

☎ CALL AN
AMBULANCE

CONTINUE GIVING
RESCUE BREATHS
UNTIL HELP
ARRIVES

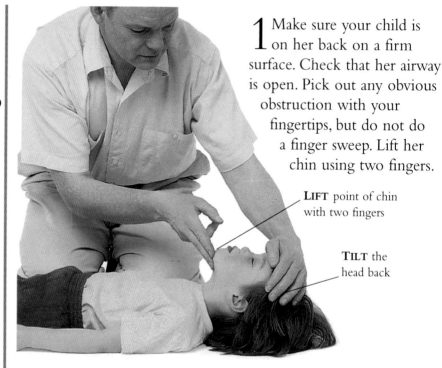

1 Make sure your child is on her back on a firm surface. Check that her airway is open. Pick out any obvious obstruction with your fingertips, but do not do a finger sweep. Lift her chin using two fingers.

LIFT point of chin with two fingers

TILT the head back

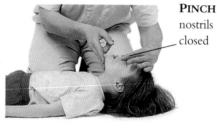

PINCH nostrils closed

2 Pinch her nostrils closed. Seal your lips round her open mouth. Breathe into the lungs until you see the chest rise.

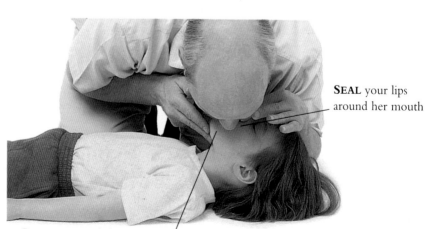

SEAL your lips around her mouth

BREATHE until the chest rises

26

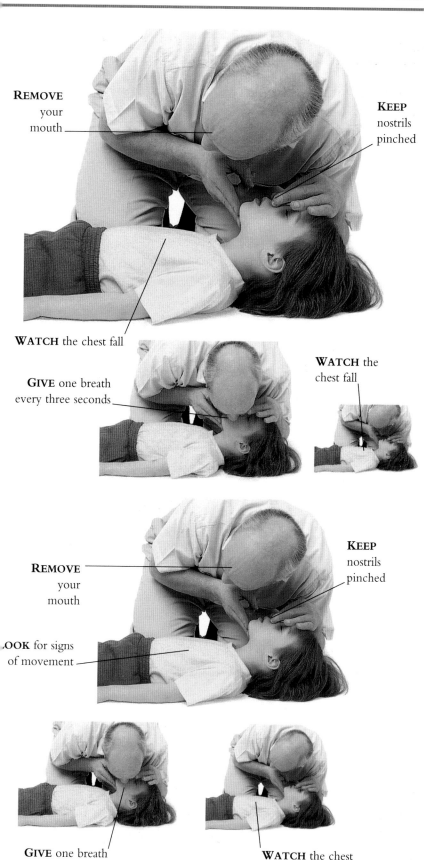

REMOVE
your
mouth

KEEP
nostrils
pinched

WATCH the chest fall

GIVE one breath
every three seconds

WATCH the
chest fall

REMOVE
your
mouth

KEEP
nostrils
pinched

LOOK for signs
of movement

GIVE one breath
every three seconds

WATCH the chest
fall after each breath

3 Remove your mouth
and let the chest fall.
Keep the nostrils pinched.
A breath is effective if the
chest rises and falls.

> **IF** *your child's chest does
> not rise, check her mouth
> again and adjust the position
> of her head.*

4 Repeat rescue breath
attempts up to five times
if necessary, to achieve two
effective breaths.

5 Stop and check for signs
of circulation (see p.22).
If these are absent, start
CPR, or cardiopulmonary
resuscitation, (see overleaf).
Otherwise, continue to give
rescue breaths for one minute,
aiming for one effective
breath every three seconds
(about 20 breaths per minute).

6 ☎ CALL AN
AMBULANCE

7 Continue to give rescue
breaths until help arrives.
Check for signs of circulation
every minute. If absent, start
CPR (see overleaf).

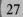

27

CPR (CARDIOPULMONARY RESUSCITATION) : CHILD

To be used for an unconscious child who is not breathing and has no signs of circulation (see p.22). Give CPR for a full minute before you call an ambulance.

RESUSCITATION SUMMARY

UNCONSCIOUS CHILD

AIRWAY OPEN

NO BREATHING

GIVE 2 EFFECTIVE RESCUE BREATHS
(see p.26)

NO SIGNS OF CIRCULATION

CPR – 5 CHEST COMPRESSIONS, 1 RESCUE BREATH – REPEATED FOR 1 MINUTE

☎ CALL AN AMBULANCE

CONTINUE **CPR** UNTIL HELP ARRIVES

28

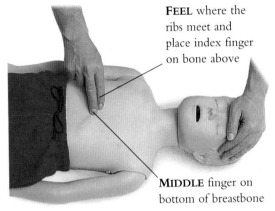

FEEL where the ribs meet and place index finger on bone above

MIDDLE finger on bottom of breastbone

1 Place your child on her back on a firm surface. Find the point on the chest where the ribs meet (breastbone). Put your middle finger on the bottom of the breastbone, your index finger on the bone above.

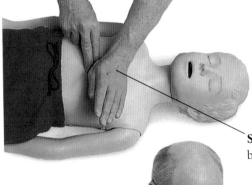

SLIDE other hand along breastbone to meet fingers

2 Slide the heel of your other hand down the breastbone to meet your fingers.

3 Using the heel of one hand only, press down sharply at this point by one-third of the depth of the chest. Do this five times at a rate of 100 compressions per minute.

PRESS down by one-third of the depth of the chest

COMPRESS chest 5 times at a rate of 100 compressions per minute

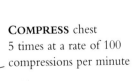

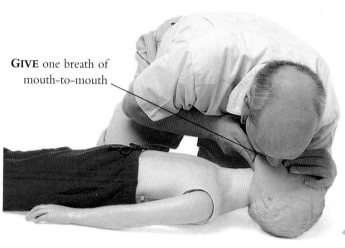

GIVE one breath of mouth-to-mouth

4 Give one rescue breath (see p.26).

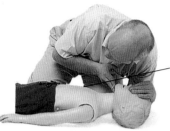

WATCH chest fall

Repeat steps 3 and 4 for about a minute

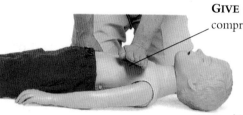

GIVE five chest compressions

5 Continue the CPR cycle of five chest compressions to one rescue breath for about a minute.

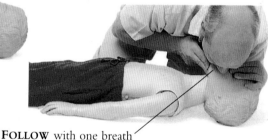

FOLLOW with one breath

Repeat CPR cycles until help arrives

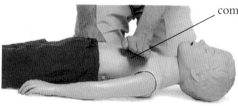

GIVE five chest compressions

6 ☎ CALL AN AMBULANCE

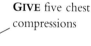

FOLLOW with one breath

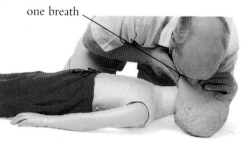

DO NOT *stop to make circulation checks unless your child makes a movement or takes a spontaneous breath. If breathing and circulation return, place your child in the* RECOVERY POSITION *(see p.24) and monitor her carefully until the ambulance arrives.*

7 Continue giving CPR – five chest compressions followed by one rescue breath – until the ambulance arrives.

29

SHOCK

Recognising shock This develops from the early signs of • *Pale, cold, and sweaty skin, tinged with grey* • *Rapid pulse becoming weaker* • *Shallow, fast breathing,* to the later signs of

• *Restlessness, yawning, and sighing* • *Thirst*
• *Loss of consciousness*

> **THE** *most likely cause of shock in a child is serious BLEEDING, see p. 46, or a SEVERE BURN OR SCALD, see p. 60. These injuries must be treated without delay.*

> **DO NOT** *give your child anything to drink or eat. If he is thirsty, moisten his lips with water.*

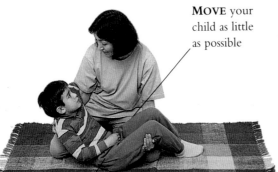

MOVE your child as little as possible

LAY him down, on blanket, coat, or rug, if possible

1 Lay your child down flat. Keep his head low as this improves the blood supply to the brain. Reassure him. Treat any injury.

☎ CALL AN AMBULANCE

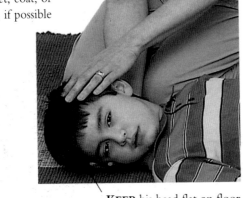

KEEP his head flat on floor

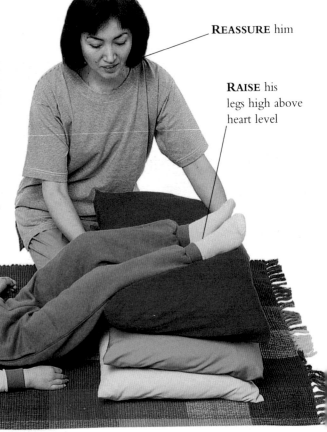

REASSURE him

RAISE his legs high above heart level

2 Carefully raise your child's legs and support them with pillows, on a chair, or on a pile of books padded with a cushion.

KEEP his head lower than his chest

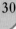
30

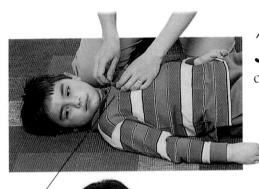

3 To make breathing easier, loosen any fastenings or tight clothing at his neck, chest, or waist.

LOOSEN any tight clothing

GIVE constant reassurance

OBSERVE his breathing rate and skin colour

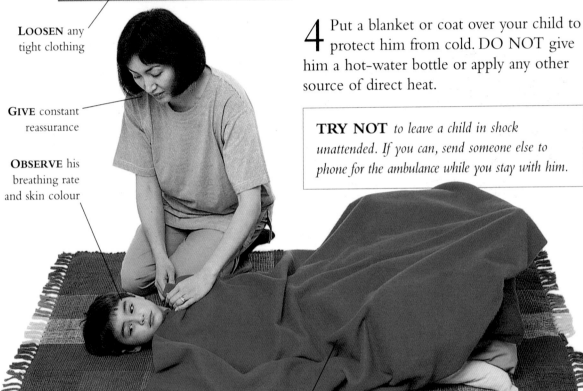

4 Put a blanket or coat over your child to protect him from cold. DO NOT give him a hot-water bottle or apply any other source of direct heat.

TRY NOT *to leave a child in shock unattended. If you can, send someone else to phone for the ambulance while you stay with him.*

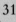

31

COVER him with a blanket to keep him warm

KEEP monitoring his pulse

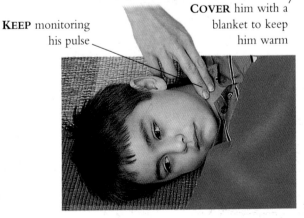

5 Keep reassuring your child. Encourage him to talk or answer questions. This will help you assess his condition. Note any changes and tell the ambulance attendant.

IF *he loses consciousness, assess his condition (see UNCONSCIOUS BABY p.16; CHILD p.22). Be prepared to resuscitate. If breathing, place him in the RECOVERY POSITION.*

FEBRILE SEIZURES

Young children may develop these seizures when they have an infection and a high temperature.

Recognising a seizure • *She may be flushed and sweating with a very hot forehead* • *Her eyes may roll upwards, be fixed or squinting* • *Her face may look blue if she is holding her breath* • *She may stiffen and arch her back* • *Her fists may clench*

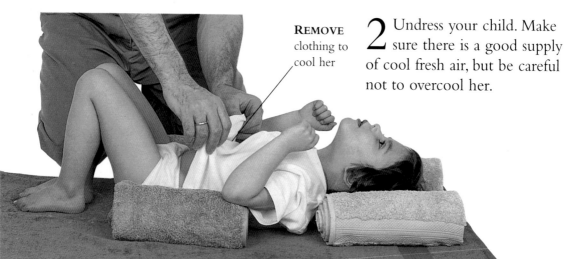

PROTECT her with padding

1 Place soft padding, such as towels or pillows, around your child so that even violent movement will not lead to injury.

REMOVE clothing to cool her

2 Undress your child. Make sure there is a good supply of cool fresh air, but be careful not to overcool her.

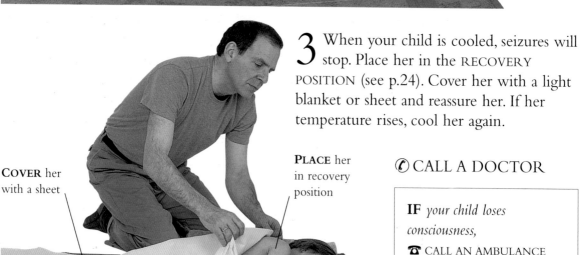

3 When your child is cooled, seizures will stop. Place her in the RECOVERY POSITION (see p.24). Cover her with a light blanket or sheet and reassure her. If her temperature rises, cool her again.

COVER her with a sheet

PLACE her in recovery position

✆ CALL A DOCTOR

IF *your child loses consciousness,*
☎ CALL AN AMBULANCE

32

EPILEPTIC SEIZURES

Recognising major epilepsy A seizure may progress through the following stages: • *Sudden falling into unconsciousness, sometimes with a cry* • *Rigidity and arching of back* • *Breathing may cease* • *Jerking movements* • *Froth or bubbles around the mouth, may be blood stained* • *Bladder or bowel control lost* • *Conscious within a few minutes* • *Dazed feeling* • *Deep sleep may follow*

Children with a history of epilepsy may have a card or bracelet alerting you to this. A child may have a minor seizure before a major one. This can be recognised by a momentary "switching off", some facial twitching, or distracted movements such as lip-smacking. If this happens, reassure the child and arrange to see your doctor.

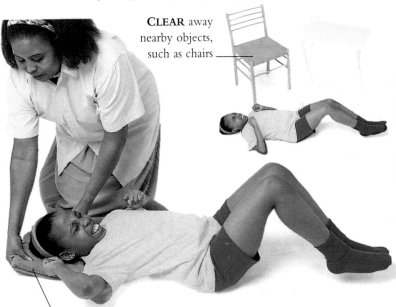

CLEAR away nearby objects, such as chairs

PROTECT her head with soft padding

1 If your child starts to fall, help her to the floor. Clear away objects that she may knock against. Place padding under or around her head. Do not hold her down or try to move her. Don't put anything in her mouth or give her anything to eat or drink.

33

Once the seizure has stopped

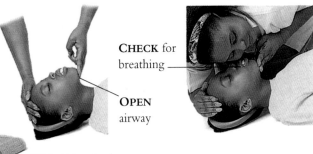

CHECK for breathing

OPEN airway

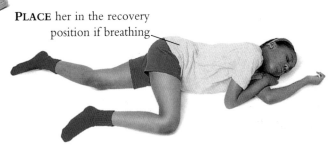

PLACE her in the recovery position if breathing

2 When her seizure is over, your child may be unconscious. Remove any padding and assess her (see p. 22). If breathing, place her in the RECOVERY POSITION (see p.24). Stay with her until she is recovered. She may feel dazed and behave oddly, or she may sleep deeply.
Ⓒ CALL A DOCTOR

IF *your child has never had a seizure before, if she has repeated seizures, or if she remains unconscious for more than ten minutes,*
☎ CALL AN AMBULANCE

DIABETIC EMERGENCY

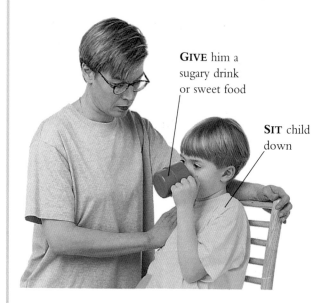

GIVE him a sugary drink or sweet food

SIT child down

Recognising low blood sugar
• *Weakness or hunger* • *Confused or aggressive behaviour* • *Sweating* • *Very pale face* • *Strong, bounding pulse* • *Shallow breathing*

> *A child who is diabetic is likely to be on insulin. Even if he seems recovered, a doctor should be asked to check the insulin dosage.*

If he improves rapidly after a sweet drink or food, give him some more and let him rest. If he does not improve,
☎ CALL AN AMBULANCE

An unconscious child

34

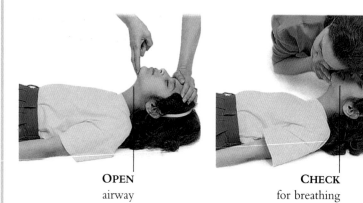

OPEN airway

CHECK for breathing

1 Open the airway and check that breathing is present.

> **IF** *your child is not breathing, be prepared to resuscitate (see UNCONSCIOUS BABY p.16; CHILD p.22).*

2 If she is breathing, place her in the RECOVERY POSITION (see p.24).

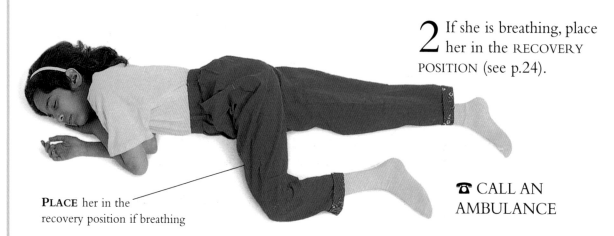

PLACE her in the recovery position if breathing

☎ CALL AN AMBULANCE

FAINT

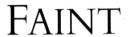

Recognising a faint • *Child feels weak, giddy and sick* • *Very pale face* • *Brief loss of consciousness* • *Slow pulse*

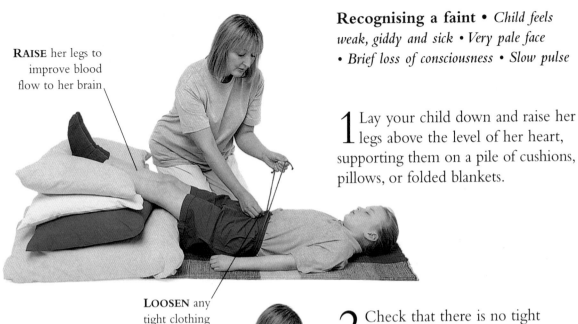

RAISE her legs to improve blood flow to her brain

1 Lay your child down and raise her legs above the level of her heart, supporting them on a pile of cushions, pillows, or folded blankets.

LOOSEN any tight clothing

2 Check that there is no tight clothing around her neck, chest, and waist. Give her plenty of fresh air – open a window, if you are indoors. It may help to fan her face.

35

COOL her by fanning her face

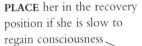

PLACE her in the recovery position if she is slow to regain consciousness

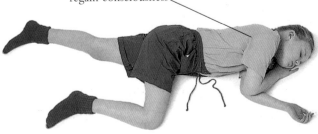

3 If your child does not regain consciousness, assess her condition (see UNCONSCIOUS BABY p.16; CHILD p.22). Be prepared to resuscitate. If breathing, place her in the RECOVERY POSITION.

☎ CALL AN AMBULANCE

CHOKING: CONSCIOUS BABY

SUMMARY

GIVE 5
BACK SLAPS

↓

CHECK MOUTH

↓

GIVE 5 CHEST
THRUSTS

↓

CHECK MOUTH

Repeat cycle of 5 back slaps, mouth check, 5 chest thrusts, mouth check, three times:

☎ CALL AN
AMBULANCE

Repeat cycle until help arrives or the obstruction clears

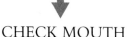

DO NOT *shake a baby*

36

Recognising a choking baby • *Breathing is obstructed* • *Trying to cry but making strange noises, or no sound* • *Face may turn blue*

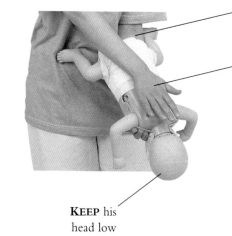

LAY him along your forearm

GIVE five sharp slaps on his back

KEEP his head low

1 Lay your baby face down with his head low along your forearm. Support his head and shoulders on your hand. Give five sharp slaps to the upper part of his back.

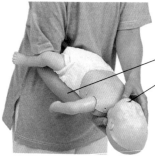

TURN HIM onto his back along your other arm

LOOK IN his mouth and remove any object you can see

2 Turn him face up along your other arm. Look inside his mouth and remove any obvious obstruction with one finger. Do not feel blindly down your baby's throat.

PLACE two fingers on breastbone, just below nipple line

GIVE five sharp downward thrusts

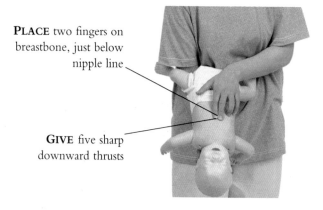

3 If back slaps fail, place two fingers on the lower half of your baby's breastbone and give five sharp downward thrusts at a rate of one every three seconds. These act as artificial coughs. Check the mouth again.

4 If the blockage hasn't cleared, repeat steps 1–3 three times. Take your baby with you and
☎ CALL AN AMBULANCE

CHOKING: UNCONSCIOUS BABY

If your baby becomes unconscious

Open the airway and check breathing (see p.16). If breathing, carefully remove any visible obstruction from the mouth. Cradle your baby in your arms with his head tilted down (see p.17).

☎ CALL AN AMBULANCE

Keep your baby in your arms and continue to check his breathing until help arrives.

SUMMARY

GIVE 2 RESCUE BREATHS

⬇

CHEST DOES NOT RISE

⬇

CPR – 5 CHEST COMPRESSIONS, 1 RESCUE BREATH FOR 1 MINUTE

⬇

☎ CALL AN AMBULANCE

Continue CPR until help arrives or the baby resumes breathing

1 If your baby is not breathing, give two effective rescue breaths (see p.18), making up to five attempts if necessary. If the chest does not rise, proceed to step 2.

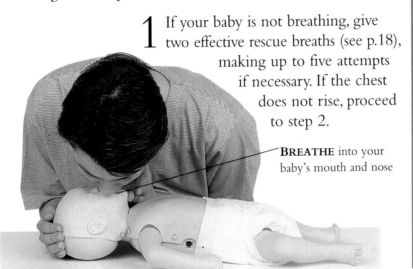

BREATHE into your baby's mouth and nose

37

2 Give five chest compressions (see CPR, p.20) in an attempt to dislodge the obstruction. Then check the mouth and give one rescue breath. Repeat CPR for one minute.

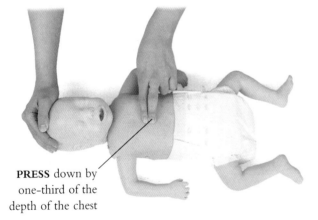

PRESS down by one-third of the depth of the chest

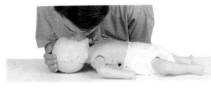

☎ CALL AN AMBULANCE

Repeat CPR cycle until help arrives

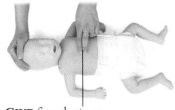

FOLLOW with one breath

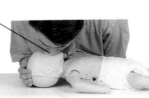

GIVE five chest compressions

3 Continue CPR until help arrives or your baby resumes breathing.

CHOKING: CONSCIOUS CHILD

SUMMARY

GIVE 5 BACK SLAPS

⬇

CHECK MOUTH

⬇

GIVE 5 CHEST
THRUSTS

⬇

CHECK MOUTH

⬇

GIVE 5 ABDOMINAL
THRUSTS

⬇

CHECK MOUTH

Repeat cycle of 5 back
slaps, mouth check, 5 chest
thrusts, mouth check, 5
adbominal thrusts, mouth
check three times

☎ CALL AN
AMBULANCE

Repeat cycle until
help arrives or the
obstruction clears

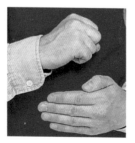

PLACE a fist against the
upper abdomen below
the rib cage.

Recognising a choking child • *Sudden clutching at the throat* • *Child unable to speak or breathe* • *Face may turn blue*

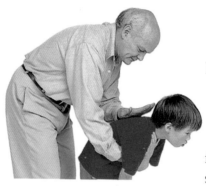

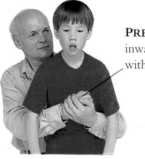

PRESS inwards with fist

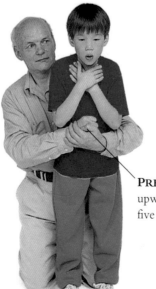

PRESS upwards five times

DO NOT *put a finger blindly down the throat*

1 Your child may be able to cough up the object on her own. Encourage her to do this, but do not waste time.

2 If this fails, make her bend forward. Give her five sharp slaps between the shoulder blades.

3 Check her mouth. Put your finger on the tongue for a clear view. Remove any object you can see.

4 If the back slaps fail, give chest thrusts. Make a fist and place it over the lower breastbone. Hold the fist with your other hand. Pull sharply *inwards* up to five times at a rate of one every three seconds. Check mouth again.

5 If the chest thrusts fail, give abdominal thrusts. Place a fist in the middle of the upper abdomen *below* the rib cage. Hold your other hand over it. Give five *upward* thrusts. Check the mouth.

6 If the abdominal thrusts fail, repeat steps 2–5 three times. If this is unsuccessful, ☎ CALL AN AMBULANCE
Continue the above cycle until help arrives or until the obstruction clears.

38

CHOKING: UNCONSCIOUS CHILD

If your child becomes unconscious

Open the airway and check breathing (see p.22). If breathing, carefully remove any visible obstruction from the mouth. Place your child in the recovery position (see p.24)

 CALL AN AMBULANCE

Keep checking his breathing until help arrives.

SUMMARY

GIVE 2 RESCUE BREATHS

⬇

CHEST DOES NOT RISE

⬇

CPR – 5 CHEST COMPRESSIONS, 1 RESCUE BREATH FOR 1 MINUTE

⬇

 CALL AN AMBULANCE

Continue CPR until help arrives or the child resumes breathing

1 If your child is not breathing, give two effective rescue breaths (see p. 26), making up to five attempts if necessary. If the chest does not rise, proceed to step 2.

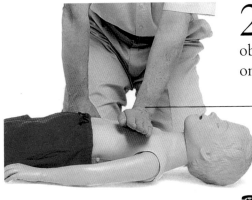

GIVE two rescue breaths

39

2 Give five chest compressions (see CPR, p.28) in an attempt to dislodge the obstruction. Then check the mouth and give one rescue breath. Repeat CPR for one minute.

COMPRESS chest five times at a rate of 100 compressions per minute

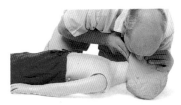

 CALL AN AMBULANCE

Repeat CPR cycle until help arrives

GIVE five chest compressions

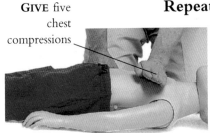

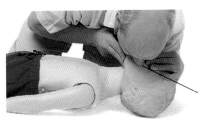

3 Continue CPR until help arrives or your child resumes breathing.

FOLLOW with one rescue breath

BREATH HOLDING

Recognising breath holding Only children under four years of age are likely to do this. • *Your child cries, breathes in but does not breathe out* • *He may go blue in the face and stiff* • *He may become unconscious momentarily*

Breath holding is the result of rage and frustration. Try to stay calm. Do not shake him or make a fuss. He will usually start breathing again spontaneously. If he loses consciousness, see UNCONSCIOUS BABY p.16; CHILD, p.22.

☎ CALL AN AMBULANCE

BLOW into his face

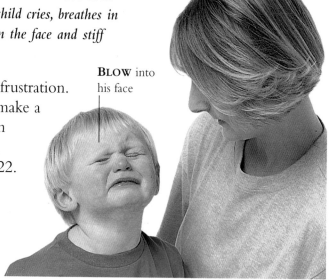

> **IF** *your baby holds his breath, blow in his face to start him breathing again.*

HICCUPS

TELL your child to sit quietly

URGE her to hold her breath for as long as possible

OR

An older child may be able to halt the attack by drinking from the wrong side of a cup.
IF *the hiccups go on for longer than a few hours,* ©CALL A DOCTOR, *as a long attack can be worrying, tiring, and painful.*

ASK her to hold a paper bag over her mouth and nose

Tell your child to sit still and to hold her breath for as long as she can. Repeat this until the hiccups have gone.
OR
Hold a paper bag over her face so that she is re-breathing her own expired air. Get her to breathe in and out for about one minute.

ENCOURAGE her to breathe in and out for one minute or until hiccups stop

SUFFOCATION

This occurs when there is an obstruction over the mouth or nose, a weight on the child's chest or abdomen preventing normal breathing, or because the child is breathing in smoke- or fume-filled air.

REMOVE
obstruction

1 Remove the obstruction as quickly as possible. This may restore breathing.

CHECK for
breathing

2 Open the airway. Place one hand on your child's forehead and gently tilt his head back. Remove any obvious obstruction from his mouth and lift his chin using two fingers. Look and listen for breathing for up to ten seconds.

OPEN airway

> **IF** *your child is not breathing, see* UNCONSCIOUS BABY *p.16;* CHILD *p.22. Be prepared to resuscitate.*

3 If he is breathing, place him in the RECOVERY POSITION (see p.24).

PLACE him in the
recovery position
if breathing

☎ CALL AN AMBULANCE Monitor the child's breathing and pulse while waiting.

41

STRANGULATION

1 Remove the constriction from around your child's neck without delay. Use scissors or a knife if necessary.

REMOVE constriction

LOOK for chest movements

> **IF** *your child is hanging, support the body while you remove the rope or cord.*

2 Open the airway. Place one hand on his forehead and gently tilt his head back. Remove any obvious obstruction from his mouth and lift his chin using two fingers.

OPEN airway

LOOK for chest movements

KEEP the head tilted back

CHECK for breathing

3 Look and listen for breathing for up to ten seconds.

> **IF** *your child is not breathing, see* UNCONSCIOUS BABY *p.16;* CHILD *p.22. Be prepared to resuscitate.*

4 If he is breathing, place him in the RECOVERY POSITION (see p.24).

☎ CALL AN AMBULANCE

Keep monitoring his breathing and pulse while you wait.

> **IF** *you suspect* BACK OR NECK INJURIES, *see pp.73–74.*

PLACE him in the recovery position if breathing

42

FUME INHALATION

Fume, gas, and smoke inhalation requires urgent medical attention.

☎ CALL AMBULANCE AND FIRE SERVICES

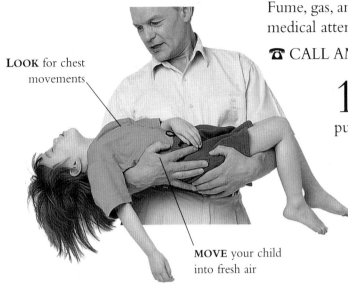

LOOK for chest movements

MOVE your child into fresh air

1 Carry your child away from the area of danger. Ensure that you do not put yourself at risk.

> IF *your child has any burns, see p.60.*

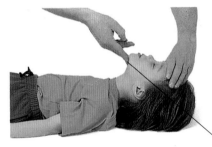

OPEN airway

2 Open the airway. Place one hand on her forehead and gently tilt her head back. Remove any obvious obstruction from her mouth and lift her chin using two fingers.

43

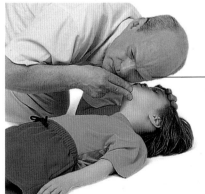

CHECK for breathing

3 Check for breathing. Feel for breath on your face and look for chest movements for up to ten seconds.

> IF *your child is not breathing, see* UNCONSCIOUS BABY *p.16;* CHILD *p.22. Be prepared to resuscitate.*

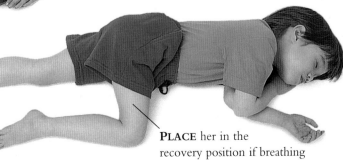

PLACE her in the recovery position if breathing

4 If your child is breathing, place her in the RECOVERY POSITION (see p.24) while you wait for help to arrive. Continue to monitor her breathing and pulse.

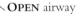

CROUP

Recognising croup This usually occurs at night. It may be alarming, but usually passes quickly. • *Difficulty breathing, particularly inhaling* • *Short, barking cough* • *Crowing or whistling noise.* In a severe attack • *Evidence that the child is using muscles around the nose, neck, and upper arms in his attempts to breathe* • *Blue-tinged skin*

SIT him up, supporting his back and head

IF *the attack is severe and affects an older child, there is a slight risk that he is suffering a rare croup-like condition called epiglottitis. Suspect epiglottitis if your child has a high temperature and is sitting bolt upright, obviously in distress.*
☎ CALL AN AMBULANCE

1 Help your child to sit up in bed. Prop him up with pillows at his back and head and reassure him.

BRING him into a steamy atmosphere to ease his breathing

KEEP your child well clear of hot running water

2 Create a steamy atmosphere; run hot water into the bath or boil a kettle in an enclosed room. Try to get your child to relax enough to breathe in the steam.

IF *the attack is severe or prolonged,*
© *CALL A DOCTOR*
Try to stay calm: if you panic this may alarm your child and worsen the attack.

ASTHMA

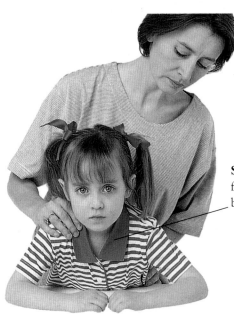

Recognising asthma • *Difficulty in breathing often accompanied by coughing* • *Wheezing on breathing out* • *Distress and anxiety* • *Tiredness from laboured breathing* • *Bluish tinge to face and lips*

1 Ensure the room is well-ventilated and smoke-free.

SIT her forward to ease breathing

IF *it is a first attack,*
℡ CALL A DOCTOR
IF *the attack is severe or does not respond to medication,*
☎ CALL AN AMBULANCE

OR

SIT her on your lap

2 Help your child to relax. Sit her down with her arms resting on a table or sit her on your lap. Reassure her as she will be frightened.

IF *your child has special medication, use it early in any attack, see below.*

45

Taking medication

If your child has medication, let him use it. Follow the directions carefully. The attack should ease. If it does not,
☎ CALL AN AMBULANCE

Various types of medication are prescribed. Familiarise your child with his medication so that he knows how to use it when he has an attack.

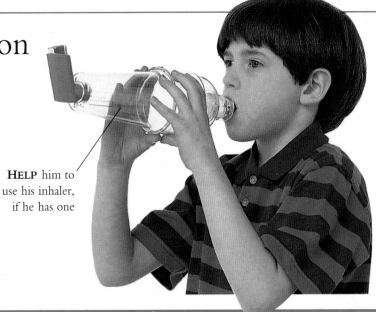

HELP him to use his inhaler, if he has one

BLEEDING

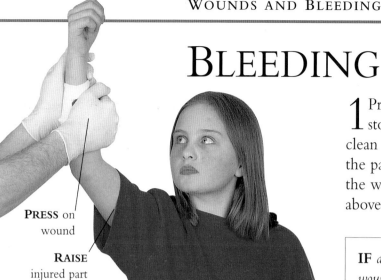

PRESS on wound

RAISE injured part

1 Press firmly on the wound to stop the bleeding. Press over a clean pad or handkerchief or put the palm of your hand directly on the wound. Raise the injured part above the level of the child's heart.

IF *an object has become stuck in the wound, see EMBEDDED OBJECT, p.48.*

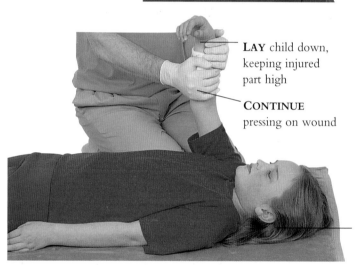

LAY child down, keeping injured part high

CONTINUE pressing on wound

2 Lay your child down, with her head low (put a thin pad under her head for comfort), and keep the injured part raised above the heart. Keep pressing on the wound for up to ten minutes.

KEEP her head low – use a thin pad for comfort

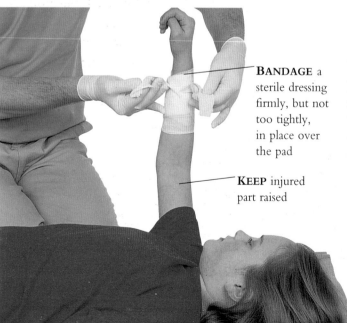

BANDAGE a sterile dressing firmly, but not too tightly, in place over the pad

KEEP injured part raised

3 Cover the wound with a sterile dressing that is larger than the wound. Bandage the dressing in place, still keeping the injured part raised. The bandage should be firm, but not so tight as to cut off the blood supply.

IF *blood comes through the bandage, bandage another pad firmly on top. If blood continues to seep through, remove both dressings and apply new ones, making sure pressure is applied over the wound.*

46

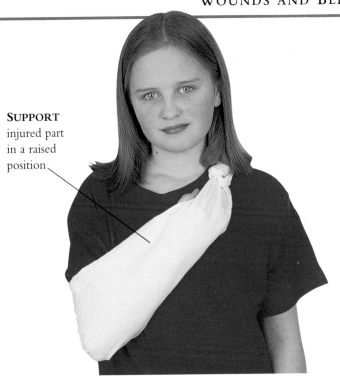

SUPPORT injured part in a raised position

4 When the bleeding is under control, support the injury – for example, with an elevation sling (see p.111).

✚ TAKE YOUR CHILD TO HOSPITAL

IF *the bleeding persists, follow the treatment for* SHOCK, *below.*
☎ CALL AN AMBULANCE

Shock

1 If the bleeding doesn't stop, raise her legs high and support them on cushions.

☎ CALL AN AMBULANCE

2 Loosen any tight clothing and, if necessary, cover her with a blanket to keep her warm. If she is thirsty, moisten her lips with water, but don't let her drink or eat. (For more on SHOCK, see pp.30–31.)

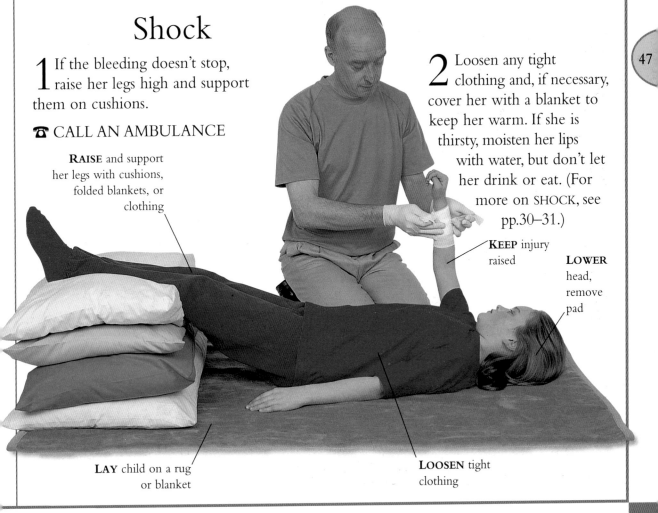

RAISE and support her legs with cushions, folded blankets, or clothing

KEEP injury raised

LOWER head, remove pad

LAY child on a rug or blanket

LOOSEN tight clothing

47

EMBEDDED OBJECT

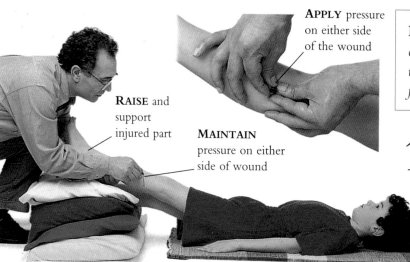

APPLY pressure on either side of the wound

RAISE and support injured part

MAINTAIN pressure on either side of wound

DO NOT *try to remove objects that are embedded in a wound as you may cause further damage and bleeding.*

1 Help your child to rest. Apply pressure on either side of the object and raise the injured part above the level of your child's heart.

DRAPE a piece of gauze over wound

2 Place a piece of gauze over the wound and object to minimise the risk of infection.

3 Use spare bandage rolls to build up padding to the same height as the embedded object.

PLACE padding around the object

4 Secure the padding by bandaging over it, being careful not to press on the embedded object.
✚ TAKE YOUR CHILD TO HOSPITAL

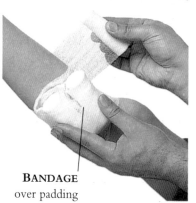

BANDAGE over padding

Bandaging around larger objects

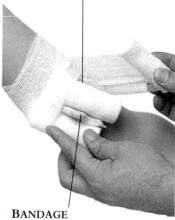

PROTECT object with pads

BANDAGE around object

IF *the object is very big, build padding around it and bandage above and below object.*

CUTS AND GRAZES

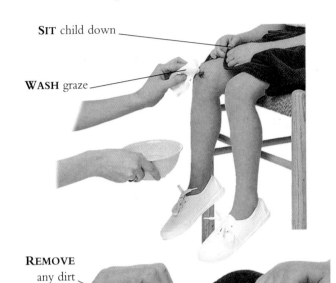

SIT child down

WASH graze

1 Sit your child down and gently wash the graze with soap and water using a gauze pad or a very soft brush.

REMOVE any dirt

2 Try to remove any particles of dirt or gravel. This may cause a little fresh bleeding.

IF *you cannot remove embedded particles of dirt,*
✚ TAKE YOUR CHILD TO HOSPITAL
Treatment will prevent a tattoo effect forming when the wound heals.

49

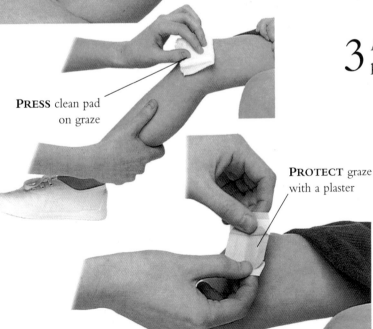

PRESS clean pad on graze

3 Apply pressure with a clean pad to stop bleeding.

PROTECT graze with a plaster

4 Dress the cut or graze with a plaster that has a pad large enough to cover the wound and the area around it.

DO NOT *cover cuts with cotton wool or any fluffy material that may stick to the wound and delay healing.*

INFECTED WOUND

Recognising an infected wound • *Increasing pain and soreness* • *Swelling, redness, and a feeling of heat around the injury* • *Pus within, or oozing from, the wound* • *Swelling and tenderness of glands in the neck, armpit, or groin* • *Faint red trails on the skin leading to these glands.* When infection is advanced • *Feverish signs of sweating, thirst, shivering, and lethargy*

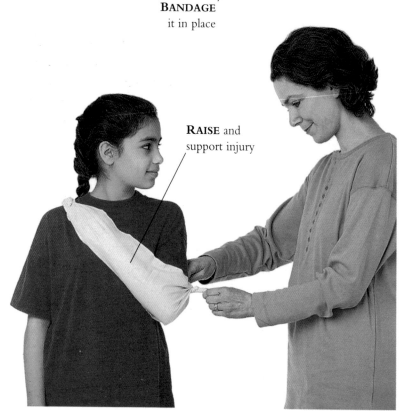

COVER
wound with
a clean pad

BANDAGE
it in place

RAISE and
support injury

1 Cover the wound with a clean non-fluffy pad or sterile dressing and then bandage it in place.

2 Raise and support the infected wound, for example with an ELEVATION SLING (see p.111).

© CALL A DOCTOR

TETANUS *is a dangerous infection that is carried in the air or in the soil. Once present in a wound, tetanus germs release toxins (poisons) into the nervous system. Tetanus is best prevented through vaccination. Babies receive this as part of their immunisation programme and a booster is given before starting school.*

50

BLISTERS

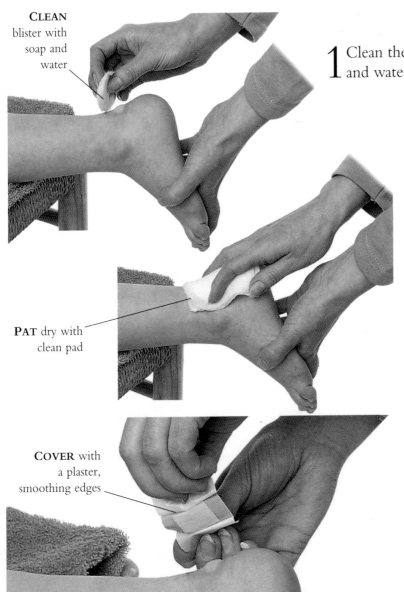

CLEAN blister with soap and water

PAT dry with clean pad

COVER with a plaster, smoothing edges

1 Clean the blister thoroughly with soap and water. Rinse it with clean water.

> **IF** *the blister has been caused by a burn, see* BURNS AND SCALDS, *p. 60.*

2 Thoroughly dry the blister and the surrounding skin. Pat it gently with a clean pad or paper tissues.

51

3 Cover the blister with a plaster. Make sure it is smooth. The plaster needs to have a pad large enough to cover the whole blister.

> **IF** *the blister is very large, cover it with a clean, non-fluffy dressing and hold it in place with adhesive tape or a bandage. Never deliberately break a blister as this can cause it to become infected.*

EYE WOUND

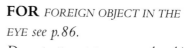

> **FOR** *FOREIGN OBJECT IN THE EYE see p.86.*
> *Do not attempt to remove the object.*
> **FOR** *CHEMICAL BURN TO THE EYE see p.64.*

1 Lay your child down and cradle his head in your lap to keep it still. Tell him to try not to move his eyes.

TELL him to keep both eyes still

LAY the child down

KEEP his head supported

2 Reassure your child and then cover the injured eye with a sterile dressing. Hold the dressing in place until you get medical help.

COVER injured eye with a sterile dressing

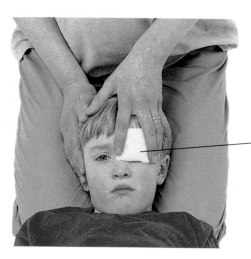

> ☎ CALL AN AMBULANCE OR
> ✚ TAKE YOUR CHILD TO HOSPITAL
> *Keep him lying on his back.*

NOSEBLEED

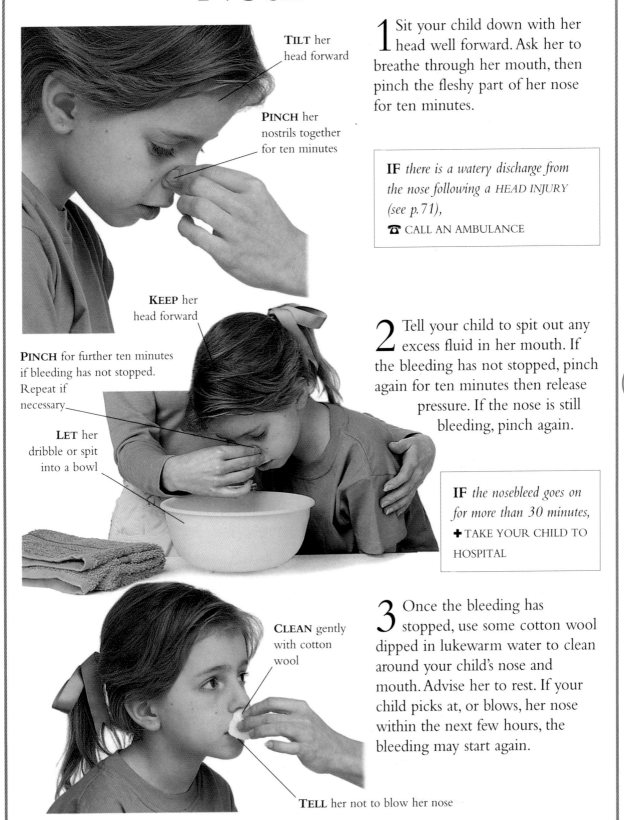

TILT her head forward

PINCH her nostrils together for ten minutes

1 Sit your child down with her head well forward. Ask her to breathe through her mouth, then pinch the fleshy part of her nose for ten minutes.

> **IF** *there is a watery discharge from the nose following a HEAD INJURY (see p.71),*
> ☎ CALL AN AMBULANCE

KEEP her head forward

PINCH for further ten minutes if bleeding has not stopped. Repeat if necessary

LET her dribble or spit into a bowl

2 Tell your child to spit out any excess fluid in her mouth. If the bleeding has not stopped, pinch again for ten minutes then release pressure. If the nose is still bleeding, pinch again.

53

> **IF** *the nosebleed goes on for more than 30 minutes,*
> ✚ TAKE YOUR CHILD TO HOSPITAL

CLEAN gently with cotton wool

3 Once the bleeding has stopped, use some cotton wool dipped in lukewarm water to clean around your child's nose and mouth. Advise her to rest. If your child picks at, or blows, her nose within the next few hours, the bleeding may start again.

TELL her not to blow her nose

EAR
Bleeding from inside the ear

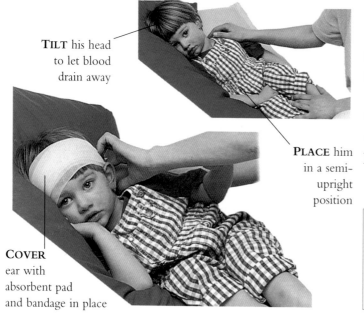

TILT his head to let blood drain away

PLACE him in a semi-upright position

COVER ear with absorbent pad and bandage in place

1 Help your child into a semi-upright position, with his head tilted towards the injured side, to allow blood to drain away.

2 Put an absorbent pad over the ear and bandage it lightly in place. Do not plug the ear.

C CALL A DOCTOR

IF *the bleeding follows a head injury (see p.71) and the fluid draining from the ear is thin and watery,*
☎ CALL AN AMBULANCE

54

External bleeding

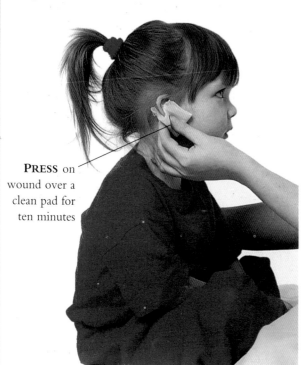

PRESS on wound over a clean pad for ten minutes

1 Gently pinch the wound with a piece of gauze, pressing for ten minutes.

2 Cover her ear with a sterile dressing and lightly bandage it in place.

C CALL A DOCTOR

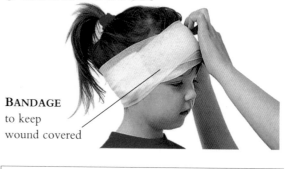

BANDAGE to keep wound covered

IF *the injury is caused by an earring being ripped out, your child may need stitches.*
✚ TAKE YOUR CHILD TO HOSPITAL

MOUTH INJURY

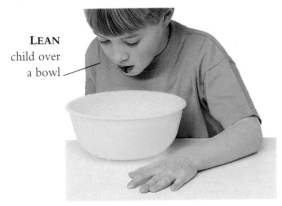

LEAN child over a bowl

DO NOT *wash out his mouth as this may disturb a blood clot.*

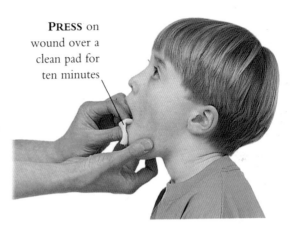

PRESS on wound over a clean pad for ten minutes

1 Sit your child down, with his head over a bowl into which he can dribble the blood.

2 Place a pad over the wound and pinch it between your thumb and forefinger, maintaining the pressure for ten minutes.

Knocked out tooth

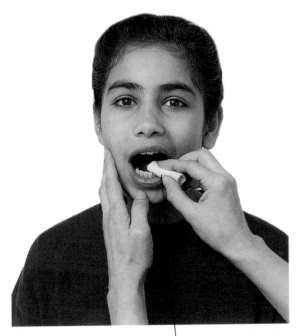

AN "ADULT" TOOTH *may be re-planted. Do not clean it. Put the tooth in milk.*
✚ TAKE YOUR CHILD TO THE DENTIST

1 Place a pad over the tooth socket, making sure that it is higher than the adjacent teeth so that your child can bite on it.

2 Ask your child to sit down with her hand supporting her jaw. Tell her to bite hard on the pad. A younger child may need you to hold the pad in place.

HOLD a pad over the tooth socket

MILK TEETH *are not re-planted, but try to find the tooth to ensure that it has not been inhaled or swallowed. A dentist should check the gum.*

55

AMPUTATION

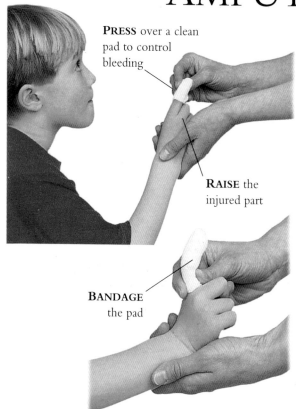

PRESS over a clean pad to control bleeding

RAISE the injured part

BANDAGE the pad

1 Control the blood loss by pressing firmly on the injury using a sterile dressing or clean pad. Raise the injured part above the level of your child's heart.

> **DO NOT** *use a tourniquet.*

2 Bandage or tape the dressing firmly in place. You can cover a finger with a gauze finger bandage.

☎ CALL AN AMBULANCE
Tell the control it is an amputation.

> **YOU** *may need to treat your child for* SHOCK, *see p.30, and* BLEEDING, *p.46.*

56

Care of the amputated part

IT *is often possible to reattach an amputated part using microsurgery. The sooner both the child and the severed part reach hospital, the better.* **NEVER** *wash the severed part or allow it to come into direct contact with the ice.* **DO NOT** *apply cotton wool to any raw surface.*

1 Wrap the severed part in kitchen film or a plastic bag.

2 Wrap the bag in a soft fabric, such as a cotton handkerchief or gauze.

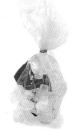

3 Put a plastic bag filled with ice cubes around the fabric. This helps preserve the severed part.

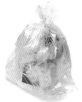

4 Put the whole package in another bag or container. Mark with the time of injury and the child's name. Give it to the ambulance attendant.

INTERNAL BLEEDING

Suspect this when signs of SHOCK (see p.30) develop without obvious blood loss.

Recognising internal bleeding • *Pale, cold, and sweaty skin tinged with grey* • *A rapid pulse becoming weaker* • *Shallow, fast breathing* • *Restlessness, yawning, and sighing* • *Thirst* • *Possible loss of consciousness.*

After violent injury, there may be: • *"Pattern bruising" at the site of injury with marks from* *clothes or crushing objects* • *Bleeding from orifices – note what it looks like and try to take a sample to hospital.*

IF *your child loses consciousness, assess her condition (see UNCONSCIOUS BABY p.16; CHILD p.22). Be prepared to resuscitate. If breathing, place her in the RECOVERY POSITION.*

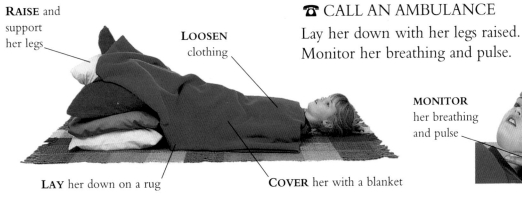

RAISE and support her legs

LOOSEN clothing

LAY her down on a rug

COVER her with a blanket

☎ CALL AN AMBULANCE

Lay her down with her legs raised. Monitor her breathing and pulse.

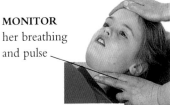

MONITOR her breathing and pulse

CRUSH INJURY

☎ CALL AN AMBULANCE

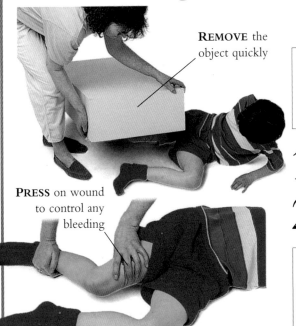

REMOVE the object quickly

PRESS on wound to control any bleeding

IF *your child has been crushed for more than 15 minutes, do not remove the object as this increases the risk of shock and further internal injury. Reassure him.*

1 If the accident has just happened, remove the heavy object quickly.

2 Control any bleeding by pressing firmly on the wound, with your hand or a clean pad.

IF *you suspect broken bones, support the injury with padding, but do not move your child until help arrives. Watch for signs of SHOCK (see above and p.30).*

57

CHEST WOUND

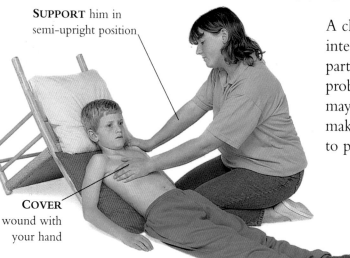

SUPPORT him in semi-upright position

COVER wound with your hand

A chest wound may cause severe internal damage. The lungs are particularly vulnerable, and breathing problems, shock, and collapsed lungs may follow an injury. It is important to make an airtight seal over the wound to prevent air entering the cavity.

PLACE clean pad over wound

COVER pad with kitchen film and secure with strapping

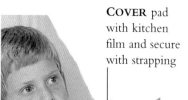

1 Cover the wound with the palm of your hand and support your child in a semi-upright position.

2 With your child supported, cover the wound with a sterile dressing or clean pad and tape it in place.

3 Create a seal over the wound with kitchen film. Secure on three sides with tape.

4 Incline your child towards his injured side, supported on cushions.

REASSURE him

TURN child to lean on injured side

IF *your child loses consciousness, assess his condition (see* UNCONSCIOUS BABY *p.16;* CHILD *p.22). Be prepared to resuscitate. If breathing, place him in the* RECOVERY POSITION *lying on his injured side. Check for signs of* SHOCK *(see p.30).*

☎ CALL AN AMBULANCE

58

ABDOMINAL WOUND

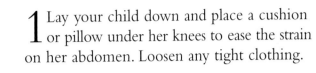

1 Lay your child down and place a cushion or pillow under her knees to ease the strain on her abdomen. Loosen any tight clothing.

BEND her knees and support her with a cushion

LAY child down gently

COVER wound with dressing

2 Reassure your child while you place a large sterile dressing over the wound. Press over the wound if your child is about to cough or vomit.

59

IF *part of the intestine is showing, cover it with a polythene bag or kitchen film before dressing the wound.*

TAPE dressing in place

3 Use adhesive tape to secure the dressing lightly in place. Continue to reassure her and watch for any change in her condition; look particularly for signs of SHOCK (p.30).

☎ CALL AN AMBULANCE

IF *your child loses consciousness, assess her condition (see UNCONSCIOUS BABY p.16; CHILD p.22). Be prepared to resuscitate.*

BURNS AND SCALDS

For information on dealing with fires, see ACTION IN AN EMERGENCY p.11.

> **DO NOT** *remove any clothing or material that may be sticking to the burned area as this may cause further damage to the skin.*

✚ TAKE YOUR CHILD TO HOSPITAL OR
☎ CALL AN AMBULANCE

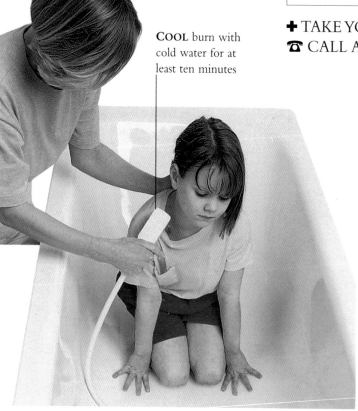

COOL burn with cold water for at least ten minutes

1 To stop the burning process and relieve pain, cool the burn with cold water for at least ten minutes.

> **IF** *no cold water is available, use another cool liquid such as milk.*

> **DO NOT** *immerse young children in cold water as this can cause hypothermia.*

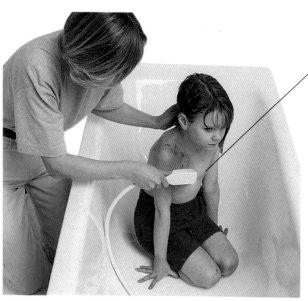

REMOVE cooled clothing and cool injury again

2 Once cooled, remove clothing from the burned area and, if the pain persists, cool again. Cut around any material that is sticking to the skin. Remove all restrictive clothing from the area of a burn before any swelling occurs.

> **DO NOT** *touch the burn or burst any blisters.*

60

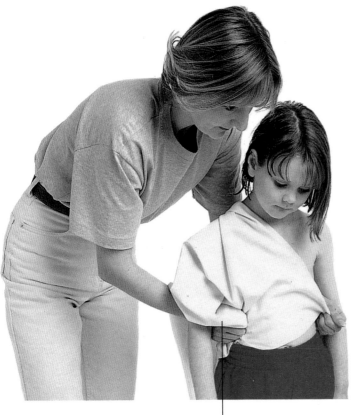

3 Cover the burn with clean, non-fluffy material to protect it from infection. You can use a clean sheet or pillow case. The dressing does not need to be secured. Do not apply lotions, fat, or ointment. Ensure that the child remains warm to prevent the onset of hypothermia.

> **DO NOT** *give her anything to eat or drink and watch for signs of SHOCK (see p.30).*

> **IF** *she loses consciousness, assess her condition (see UNCONSCIOUS BABY p.16; CHILD p.22). Be prepared to resuscitate. If breathing, place her in the RECOVERY POSITION.*

COVER burn loosely with clean, non-fluffy material

Alternative dressings

To dress a burned hand or foot you can use a plastic bag or clean kitchen film, both of which will protect the burn from infection. Secure the bag with a bandage or plaster around the bag, not the skin.

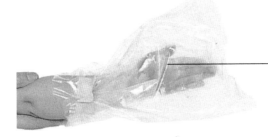

PROTECT with clean plastic bag

Burns to the mouth and throat

Burns in this area are very serious as they cause swelling and inflammation of the air passages, giving a serious risk of suffocation. Act quickly. If necessary, loosen clothing from around his neck.

☎ CALL AN AMBULANCE

> **IF** *your child develops breathing difficulties, assess his condition (see UNCONSCIOUS BABY p.16; CHILD p.22). Be prepared to resuscitate.*

61

ELECTRICAL BURN

An electric shock from a low-voltage source can result in burns. These may occur at both the point of entry and the point of exit of an electrical current. See ELECTRICAL INJURY (p.12), SHOCK (p.30).

DO NOT *touch your child directly until you are sure the electrical current is switched off.*

IF *your child loses consciousness, assess her condition (see UNCONSCIOUS BABY p.16; CHILD p.22). Be prepared to resuscitate. If breathing, place her in the RECOVERY POSITION.*

COOL burns with cold water for at least ten minutes

1 Hold the injured area under cold, running water for at least ten minutes to cool the burn.

2 Protect the burn by covering it with clean, non-fluffy material or with a plastic bag, held or taped in place.

+ TAKE YOUR CHILD TO HOSPITAL

COVER with a clean plastic bag

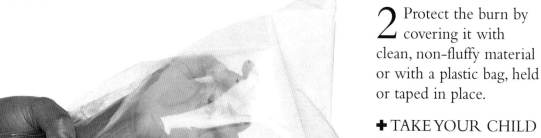

CHEMICAL BURN TO SKIN

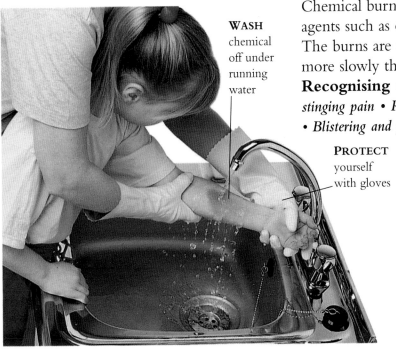

WASH chemical off under running water

PROTECT yourself with gloves

Chemical burns can be caused by household agents such as oven cleaner or paint stripper. The burns are serious but signs develop more slowly than for thermal burns.
Recognising chemical burns • *Fierce, stinging pain* • *Redness or staining*, followed by • *Blistering and peeling*

1 Wash away all traces of the chemical by holding the affected area under plenty of running water.

NOTE *the name of the substance that caused the burn. Wear protective rubber gloves, and beware of fumes. See FUME INHALATION p. 43, and SWALLOWED CHEMICALS p. 65.*

63

Removing clothes

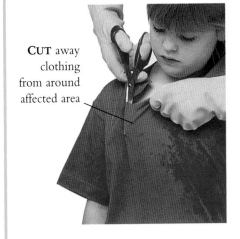

CUT away clothing from around affected area

COVER burn loosely with clean, non-fluffy material

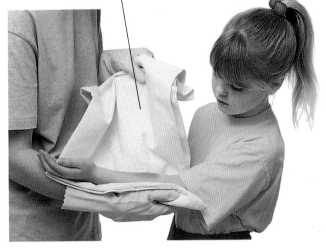

Cut off clothing from the affected area, unless you can slip it off without touching other parts of the body. Avoid cutting through the affected area – cut around it instead.

2 Loosely cover the burn with clean, non-fluffy material, such as a pillow case. This avoids constriction when the wound swells. You can wet the pillow case to cool and soothe the burn.

✚ TAKE YOUR CHILD TO HOSPITAL

CHEMICAL BURN TO EYE

Splashes of chemicals in the eye can cause scarring or can even cause blindness.

Recognising chemical burns to the eye • *Fierce pain in the eye* • *Difficulty opening the eye* • *Redness and swelling in and around the eye* • *Very watery eye*

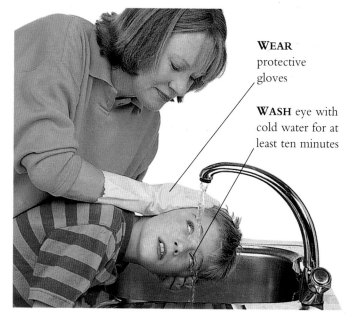

WEAR protective gloves

WASH eye with cold water for at least ten minutes

DO NOT *let your child touch his eye.*

THE EYE *will be shut in spasm and pain, so gently pull the eyelids open.*

1 Hold your child's head over a basin, with the "good" eye uppermost, and gently run cold water over the contaminated eye for at least ten minutes. Wear protective gloves. Make sure that both sides of the eyelid are thoroughly washed and that the water drains away from his face.

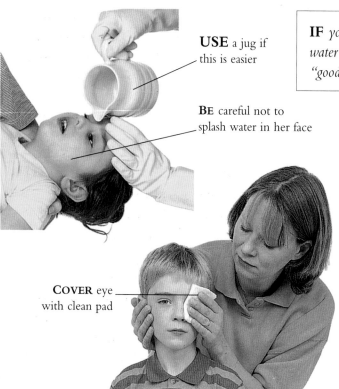

USE a jug if this is easier

BE careful not to splash water in her face

IF *you find it easier, you can use a jug to pour water over the affected eye. Avoid splashing the "good" eye with contaminated water.*

2 When the injured eye is thoroughly washed, cover it with a large sterile dressing. Hold the dressing in place until you get medical aid.

COVER eye with clean pad

✚ TAKE YOUR CHILD TO HOSPITAL

OR

☎ CALL AN AMBULANCE

64

SWALLOWED CHEMICALS

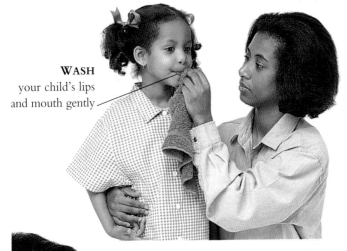

WASH your child's lips and mouth gently

IF *you think your child has swallowed anything poisonous,* ⓒ CALL A DOCTOR

1 Wipe away any residual chemical around the mouth and face.

2 Her lips may be burned or discoloured, so give her frequent sips of cold water or milk.

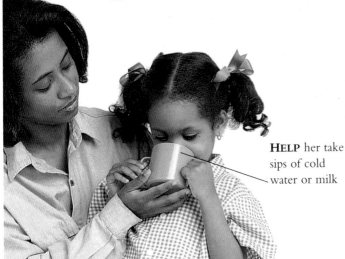

HELP her take sips of cold water or milk

DO NOT *try to make your child vomit as this can cause further harm.*

65

3 Find out what chemical your child swallowed and telephone a doctor with the information. This will help determine the correct medical treatment.

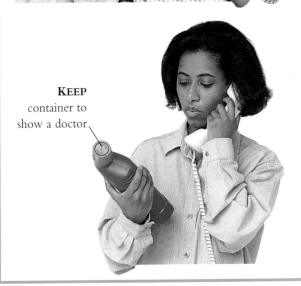

KEEP container to show a doctor

IF *your child loses consciousness, assess her condition (see* UNCONSCIOUS BABY, *p.16;* CHILD *p.22). Be prepared to resuscitate. If breathing, place her in the* RECOVERY POSITION.

DRUG POISONING

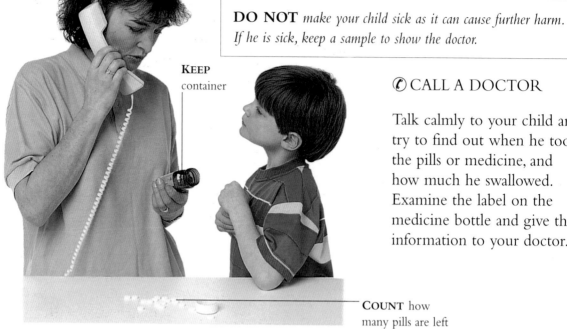

DO NOT *make your child sick as it can cause further harm. If he is sick, keep a sample to show the doctor.*

KEEP container

✆ CALL A DOCTOR

Talk calmly to your child and try to find out when he took the pills or medicine, and how much he swallowed. Examine the label on the medicine bottle and give the information to your doctor.

COUNT how many pills are left

If the child is unconscious

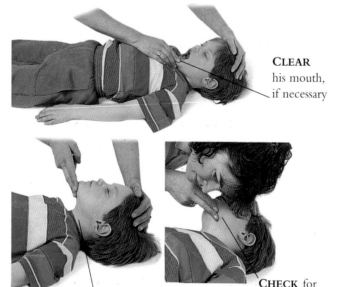

CLEAR his mouth, if necessary

☎ CALL AN AMBULANCE

1 Open his mouth. Pick out any drugs that you can see.

TRY *to find out what drugs he has taken and how much he has swallowed.*

2 Open his airway. Check his breathing (see UNCONSCIOUS BABY p.16; CHILD p.22). Be prepared to resuscitate. If he is breathing, place him in the RECOVERY POSITION. Stay with him until help arrives.

CHECK for breathing

OPEN airway

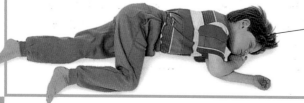

PLACE him in recovery position if breathing

66

ALCOHOL POISONING

EVEN *a small amount of alcohol may harm a young child.*

Recognising alcohol poisoning
- Strong smell of alcohol • Flushed and moist face • Slurred speech
- Staggering • Deep noisy breathing
- Nausea • Bounding pulse

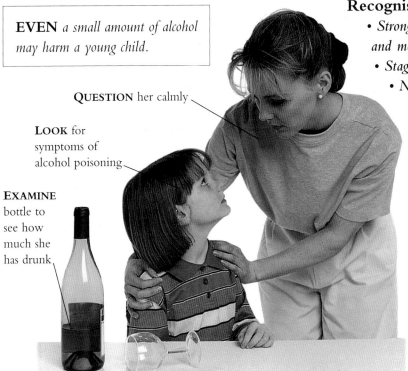

QUESTION her calmly

LOOK for symptoms of alcohol poisoning

EXAMINE bottle to see how much she has drunk

✆ CALL A DOCTOR

Allow your child to rest where you can watch over her. Place a bowl nearby in case she is sick. If she falls asleep, check her to make sure she can be easily roused. If she is very drowsy, or seems unconscious, see below.

67

If the child is unconscious

☎ CALL AN AMBULANCE

KEEP *your child warm. Alcohol dilates the blood vessels, which can cause hypothermia.*

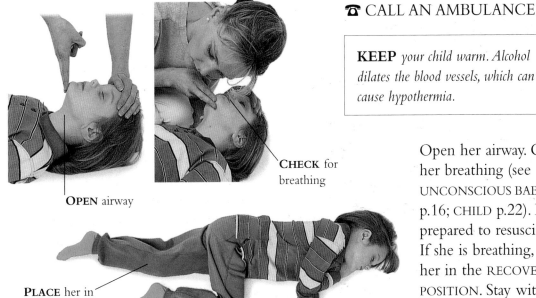

OPEN airway

CHECK for breathing

PLACE her in recovery position if breathing

Open her airway. Check her breathing (see UNCONSCIOUS BABY p.16; CHILD p.22). Be prepared to resuscitate. If she is breathing, place her in the RECOVERY POSITION. Stay with her until help arrives.

PLANT POISONING

ASK him how much he ate

1 Try to find out what your child has eaten and keep a sample to show the doctor.
Ⓒ CALL A DOCTOR

> **DO NOT** *make your child sick. This can cause further harm. If he is sick, show a sample to the doctor.*

2 Look inside your child's mouth. Pick out any remaining pieces of plant or berries.

KEEP piece of plant or any berries to show doctor

REMOVE any residue

If the child is unconscious

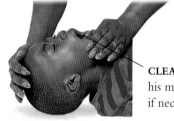

1 Open his mouth. Pick out any pieces of plant that you can see.
☎ CALL AN AMBULANCE

CLEAR his mouth, if necessary

2 Open his airway. Check his breathing (see UNCONSCIOUS BABY p.16; CHILD p.22). Be prepared to resuscitate.

CHECK for breathing

OPEN airway

> **IF** *he is breathing, place him in the* RECOVERY POSITION. *Stay with him until the ambulance arrives.*

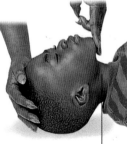
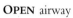

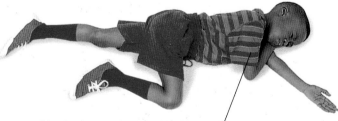

PLACE him in recovery position if breathing

SCALP WOUND

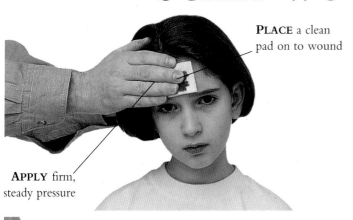

PLACE a clean pad on to wound

APPLY firm, steady pressure

1 Cover the injury with a clean pad or sterile dressing that is larger than the wound. Press firmly on the pad and the wound to control the bleeding. Place another pad on top, if necessary, and keep pressing on the wound. If blood continues to seep through, remove both pads and apply new ones.

BANDAGE pad in place

SECURE bandage firmly but not too tightly

2 Bandage the dressing firmly in place. If the bleeding continues, apply pressure again with your hand.

> **IF** *the wound has been caused by a blow to the head,*
> ℂ CALL A DOCTOR
> *(see also CONCUSSION p. 70; SKULL FRACTURE p. 71).*

69

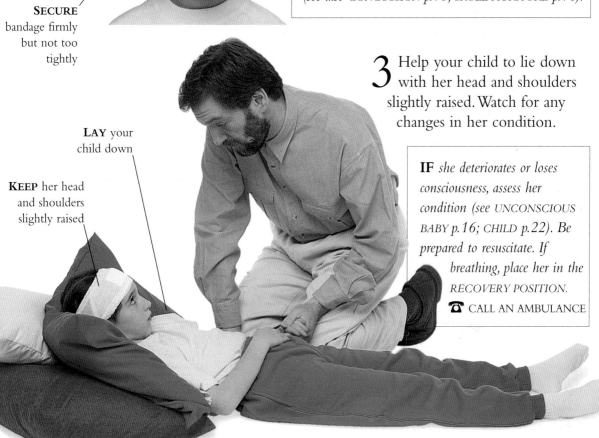

LAY your child down

KEEP her head and shoulders slightly raised

3 Help your child to lie down with her head and shoulders slightly raised. Watch for any changes in her condition.

> **IF** *she deteriorates or loses consciousness, assess her condition (see UNCONSCIOUS BABY p. 16; CHILD p. 22). Be prepared to resuscitate. If breathing, place her in the RECOVERY POSITION.*
> ☎ CALL AN AMBULANCE

CONCUSSION

The brain may be "shaken" by a blow causing concussion. The period of unconsciousness is brief and followed by complete recovery. You should be able to distinguish between a bump on the head with no concussion, a brief period of concussion (less than 20 seconds), and an extended period of unconsciousness.

Recognising concussion • *Brief loss of consciousness, dizziness or nausea on recovery* • *Loss of memory of immediately preceding events* • *A mild headache*

Conscious child

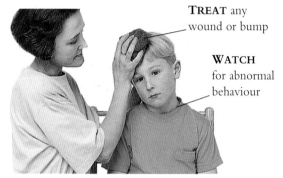

TREAT any wound or bump

WATCH for abnormal behaviour

If your child has bumped his head, sit him down and treat any minor bruise or wound with a cold compress.

> **WATCH** *for signs of abnormal behaviour. If he does not recover fully within a few minutes,* ℃ CALL A DOCTOR

Child who regains consciousness quickly

1 If your child has been "knocked out", even briefly,
℃ CALL A DOCTOR

2 Make her rest and watch her closely. If she does not recover completely within 30 minutes,
☎ CALL AN AMBULANCE

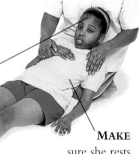

WATCH child carefully for abnormal behaviour

MAKE sure she rests

Unconscious child

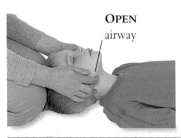

OPEN airway

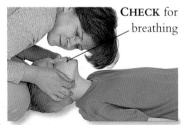

CHECK for breathing

☎ CALL AN AMBULANCE

Open your child's airway using the jaw thrust technique (see p.74). Check his breathing (see UNCONSCIOUS BABY p.16; CHILD p.22). Be prepared to resuscitate. If he is breathing, continue to support his head until help arrives. If you cannot maintain an open airway, place him in the RECOVERY POSITION (see p.24).

> **IF** *you are alone and you need to leave your child to call an ambulance, and if your child remains unconscious, place him in the RECOVERY POSITION (see p.24) before you leave.*

70

SKULL FRACTURE

Fractures of the skull are potentially very serious injuries and require urgent medical attention to minimise the risk of damage to the brain and the possibility of infection.

Recognising a skull fracture • *Wound or bruise on the head* • *Soft area on the scalp* • *Impaired consciousness* • *Deterioration in level of response* • *Clear fluid from the nose or ear*

• *Blood showing in the white of the eye*
• *Distortion of the head or face*

☎ CALL AN AMBULANCE

> **IF** *you suspect BACK or NECK INJURIES, see pp. 73–74.*

Unconscious child

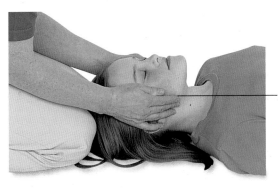

LIFT your child's jaw up with your fingertips

1 Open your child's airway using the jaw thrust technique (see p.74).

> **IF** *you are alone and you need to leave your child to call an ambulance, and if your child remains unconscious, place her in the RECOVERY POSITION (see p.24) before you leave.*

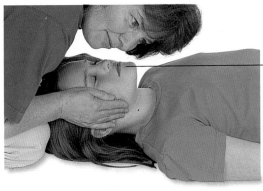

CHECK for breathing

2 Check her breathing (see UNCONSCIOUS BABY p.16; CHILD p.22). Be prepared to resuscitate. If your child is breathing, continue to support her head until help arrives. If you cannot maintain an open airway, place her in the RECOVERY POSITION (see p.24).

Delayed reaction

There may be a serious reaction to a head injury hours or even days later. Cerebral compression is a condition caused by blood accumulating within the skull and putting pressure on the brain.

Recognising cerebral compression
• *Disorientation and confusion* • *Severe headache*

• *Impaired consciousness* • *Noisy breathing, becoming slow* • *Slow but strong pulse* • *Unequal pupils* • *Weakness or paralysis* • *Raised temperature*

Be prepared to resuscitate (see UNCONSCIOUS BABY p.16; CHILD, p.22).

☎ CALL AN AMBULANCE

71

BROKEN NOSE/CHEEKBONE

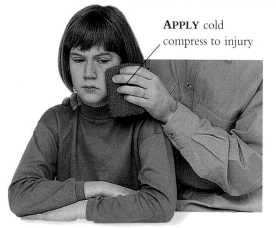

APPLY cold compress to injury

1 Sit your child down and apply a cold compress to the injured part. This helps to reduce the swelling. Hold the compress in place for about 30 minutes.

2 If your child's nose is bleeding heavily, ask her to sit with her head over a bowl and to pinch her nostrils together.

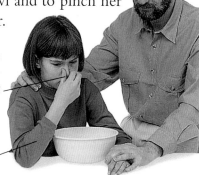

PINCH nostrils together to stop bleeding

SIT your child well forward over bowl

IF *pinching her nose hurts too much, simply ask her to sit forward and give her a soft pad or towel to soak up the blood.*

✚ TAKE YOUR CHILD TO HOSPITAL

BROKEN JAW

Recognising a broken jaw
• *Tender, swollen, bruised jaw* • *Teeth may be out of line*

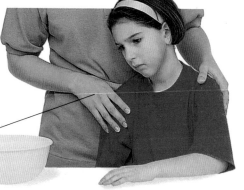

HELP her to lean forward

1 Sit her down with her head well forward. Tell her not to swallow, but to let any blood or saliva drain away.

HOLD pad against jaw and support jaw with your hand

IF *she loses consciousness, assess her condition (see UNCONSCIOUS BABY, p.16; CHILD p.22). Be prepared to resuscitate. If breathing, place her in the RECOVERY POSITION.*

☎ CALL AN AMBULANCE

2 Make a soft pad and hold it firmly under her injured jaw. Do not bandage the pad in place in case she is sick. Continue to support the jaw on the way to the hospital.

✚ TAKE YOUR CHILD TO HOSPITAL

BACK AND NECK INJURIES
The conscious child

☎ CALL AN AMBULANCE

> **DO NOT** *move the injured child unless his life is in danger.* **IF** *you do have to move him, try to do so in "one piece", taking care not to twist or bend the neck or spine.*

LEAVE a slight gap so that your child can hear you

HOLD his head in your hands

KEEP his back straight

1 Reassure your child and tell him not to move. Steady and support his head and neck by placing your hands over his ears and keeping his head in line with his spine. Be careful not to pull on his neck.

MAINTAIN support of his head

73

2 Keep his head supported in this position until help arrives. Ask someone to put rolled blankets or towels around his neck and shoulders for extra support.

PLACE rolled blankets around his head and shoulders

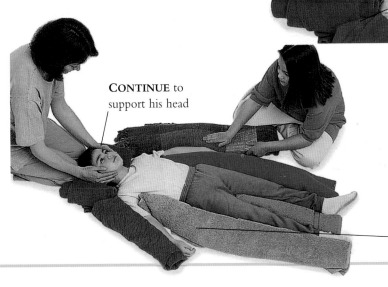

CONTINUE to support his head

3 Get a helper to arrange rolled towels or blankets around your child's neck and shoulders and either side of his body while you continue to keep his head steady.

PLACE folded blankets or towels either side of his body

BACK AND NECK INJURIES
The unconscious child

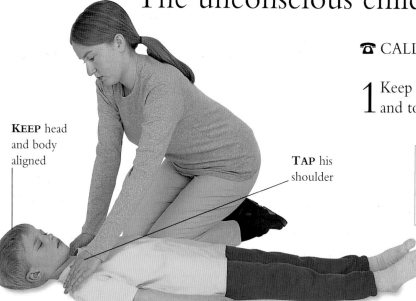

KEEP head and body aligned

TAP his shoulder

☎ CALL AN AMBULANCE

1 Keep your child's head, trunk, and toes in a straight line.

> **DO NOT MOVE**
> *your child unless his life is in immediate danger.*

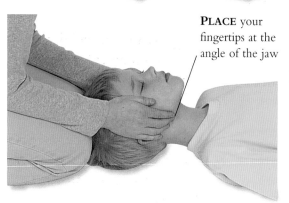

PLACE your fingertips at the angle of the jaw

2 Use the jaw thrust method to open your child's airway. Kneel behind his head and place your hands on both sides of his face, with your fingertips at the angles of his jaw. Gently lift his jaw to open the airway, taking care not to tilt his head back.

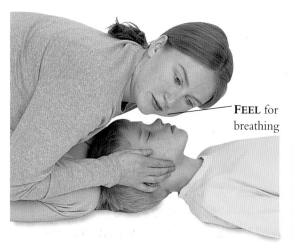

FEEL for breathing

3 Check his breathing (see UNCONSCIOUS BABY p.16; CHILD p.22). Be prepared to resuscitate. If your child is breathing, continue to support his head until help arrives. If you cannot maintain an open airway, place him in the RECOVERY POSITION (see opposite).

> **IF** *you are alone and need to leave your child to call an ambulance, and if your child remains unconscious, place him in the RECOVERY POSITION (see p.24) before you leave.*

74

Recovery position with one helper

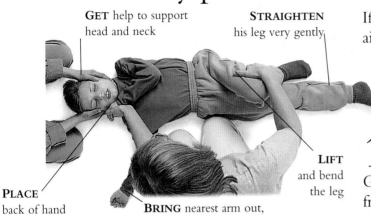

GET help to support head and neck

STRAIGHTEN his leg very gently

PLACE back of hand against his cheek

BRING nearest arm out, elbow bent, palm uppermost

LIFT and bend the leg

If you cannot maintain an open airway, for example if your child vomits, place him in the recovery position. See p.24 if you have no helper.

1 Ask the helper to support your child's head with her hands. Grasp the thigh of the leg furthest from you. Gently lift and bend the leg. Draw the arm furthest from you across the child's chest.

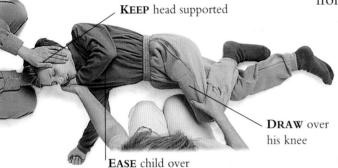

KEEP head supported

EASE child over

DRAW over his knee

2 Draw over his knee and ease him round gently. Keep his head and trunk aligned at all times.

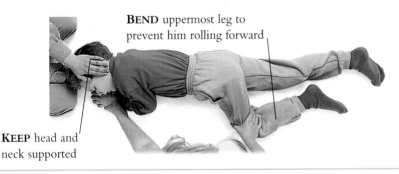

BEND uppermost leg to prevent him rolling forward

KEEP head and neck supported

3 With your child turned onto his side, maintain an open airway and support him in this position until help arrives. Monitor his breathing and pulse. Be prepared to resuscitate (see UNCONSCIOUS BABY p.16; CHILD p.22).

75

Log-roll technique

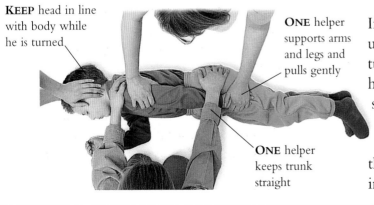

KEEP head in line with body while he is turned

ONE helper supports arms and legs and pulls gently

ONE helper keeps trunk straight

If you have two or more helpers, use the "log-roll" technique to turn your child. It is vital to keep his head, trunk and feet in a straight line. While one adult holds the child's head, two others should gently straighten the limbs and roll the child over in one synchronised movement.

BROKEN LEG

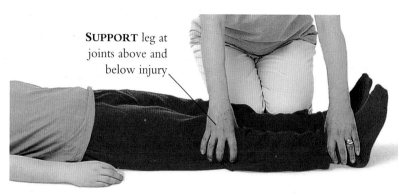

SUPPORT leg at joints above and below injury

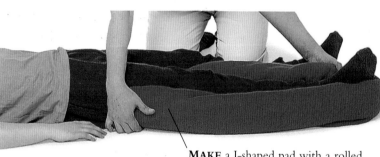

MAKE a J-shaped pad with a rolled blanket and place it around his leg

1 Lay your child down gently and support his leg at the ankle and knee joints. Ask someone to help you, if possible.

2 Steady the injured leg with padding. Pad outside the injured limb and between the legs with one or more rolled-up blankets. If necessary, cover your child with another blanket to keep him warm.

☎ CALL AN AMBULANCE

76

Making broad-fold and narrow-fold bandages

TAKE a triangular bandage

FOLD top point over to touch the base

BROAD-FOLD BANDAGE

FOLD bandage in half to make a broad-fold

NARROW-FOLD BANDAGE

FOLD bandage in half again to make a narrow-fold bandage

Tying a reef knot

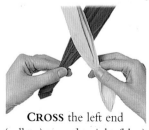

CROSS the left end (yellow) over the right (blue)

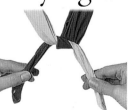

TAKE the yellow under and through

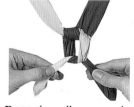

PASS the yellow over the blue and through the gap

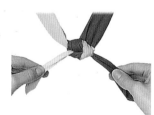

PULL the ends firmly

How to splint an injured leg

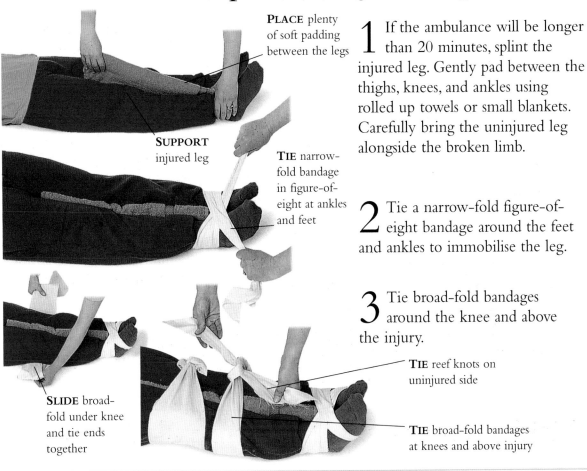

PLACE plenty of soft padding between the legs

SUPPORT injured leg

TIE narrow-fold bandage in figure-of-eight at ankles and feet

SLIDE broad-fold under knee and tie ends together

1 If the ambulance will be longer than 20 minutes, splint the injured leg. Gently pad between the thighs, knees, and ankles using rolled up towels or small blankets. Carefully bring the uninjured leg alongside the broken limb.

2 Tie a narrow-fold figure-of-eight bandage around the feet and ankles to immobilise the leg.

3 Tie broad-fold bandages around the knee and above the injury.

TIE reef knots on uninjured side

TIE broad-fold bandages at knees and above injury

77

BROKEN PELVIS

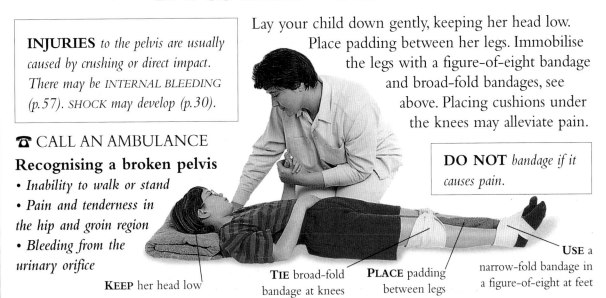

INJURIES *to the pelvis are usually caused by crushing or direct impact. There may be* INTERNAL BLEEDING *(p.57).* SHOCK *may develop (p.30).*

☎ CALL AN AMBULANCE

Recognising a broken pelvis
• *Inability to walk or stand*
• *Pain and tenderness in the hip and groin region*
• *Bleeding from the urinary orifice*

Lay your child down gently, keeping her head low. Place padding between her legs. Immobilise the legs with a figure-of-eight bandage and broad-fold bandages, see above. Placing cushions under the knees may alleviate pain.

DO NOT *bandage if it causes pain.*

KEEP her head low

TIE broad-fold bandage at knees

PLACE padding between legs

USE a narrow-fold bandage in a figure-of-eight at feet

KNEE INJURY

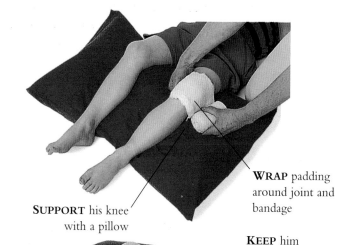

1 Help your child to lie down, then slide a pillow under the injured knee to provide support. Pad around the injured knee with cotton wool or a soft dressing.

2 Use a roller bandage to keep the padding in place, working from the child's injured side.

WRAP padding around joint and bandage

SUPPORT his knee with a pillow

> **DO NOT** *attempt to force the knee straight as this may cause further injury.*

KEEP him comfortable

> **DO NOT** *allow the child to eat, drink, or walk.*

✚ TAKE YOUR CHILD TO HOSPITAL
OR ☎ CALL AN AMBULANCE

78

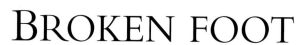

BROKEN FOOT

Fractures of the foot are usually caused by crushing.
Recognising a broken foot
• *Bruising and swelling* • *Stiffness*
• *Difficulty in walking*

Sit your child down. Raise and support the injured foot. Hold an icepack against the injury. Bandage it in place to relieve pain.

✚ TAKE YOUR CHILD TO HOSPITAL

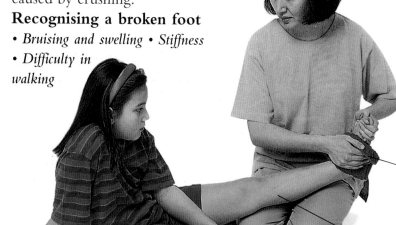

REDUCE swelling with an ice pack

KEEP leg elevated

SPRAINED ANKLE

Suspect an ankle sprain if your child can't take her full weight on her foot after a fall or wrench.

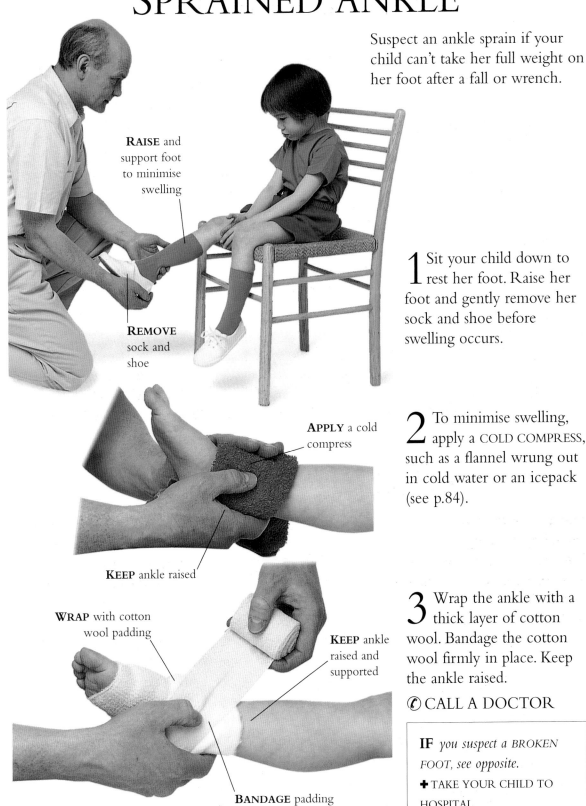

RAISE and support foot to minimise swelling

REMOVE sock and shoe

APPLY a cold compress

KEEP ankle raised

WRAP with cotton wool padding

KEEP ankle raised and supported

BANDAGE padding firmly in place

1 Sit your child down to rest her foot. Raise her foot and gently remove her sock and shoe before swelling occurs.

2 To minimise swelling, apply a COLD COMPRESS, such as a flannel wrung out in cold water or an icepack (see p.84).

3 Wrap the ankle with a thick layer of cotton wool. Bandage the cotton wool firmly in place. Keep the ankle raised.

☎ CALL A DOCTOR

> **IF** *you suspect a* BROKEN FOOT, *see opposite.*
> ✚ TAKE YOUR CHILD TO HOSPITAL

79

BROKEN COLLAR BONE

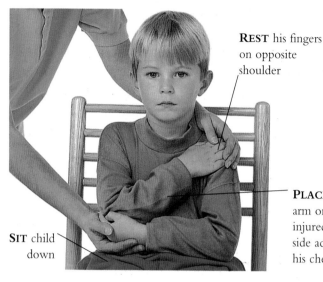

REST his fingers on opposite shoulder

PLACE arm on injured side across his chest

SIT child down

The collar bone may be broken by indirect force, if a child falls onto his outstretched hand, or by a blow to his shoulder.

Recognising a broken collar bone • *Pain and tenderness increased by movement* • *Head turned and inclined to the injured side*

1 Sit your child down and gently bring the arm on the injured side across his chest. Ask him to support his elbow in his hand.

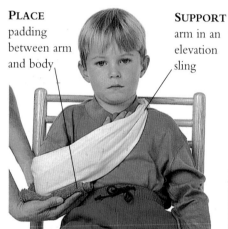

PLACE padding between arm and body

SUPPORT arm in an elevation sling

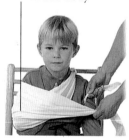

TIE a broad-fold bandage around arm and body

2 Place your child's arm in an ELEVATION SLING for support (see p.111). Use a REEF KNOT (see p.76).

3 Secure the arm with a BROAD-FOLD BANDAGE (see p.76 and below).

✚ TAKE YOUR CHILD TO HOSPITAL

Tying a broad-fold bandage around a sling

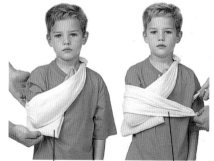

SLIDE padding between arm and body

PLACE a broad-fold bandage around body and arm

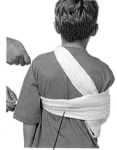

SECURE with a reef knot tied on uninjured side

A sling will support an injured arm, but a broad-fold bandage provides extra support if you need to take your child on a journey.

BROKEN RIBS

SIT your child down

SUPPORT arm on injured side in an arm sling

Recognising broken ribs • *Child has had a blow to chest, a heavy fall, or has been crushed* • *Sharp pain at the fracture site* • *Pain on breathing* • *Signs of internal bleeding* • *Open wound over the fracture site*

Support the arm on the injured side in an ARM SLING (see p.110).

✚ TAKE YOUR CHILD TO HOSPITAL

> **IF** *the child has a CHEST WOUND (see p.58) or INTERNAL BLEEDING (see p.57),*
> ☎ CALL AN AMBULANCE

Open or multiple rib fractures

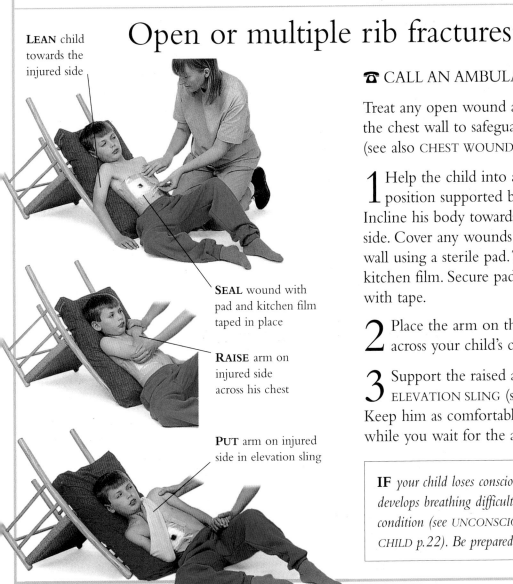

LEAN child towards the injured side

SEAL wound with pad and kitchen film taped in place

RAISE arm on injured side across his chest

PUT arm on injured side in elevation sling

☎ CALL AN AMBULANCE

Treat any open wound and support the chest wall to safeguard breathing (see also CHEST WOUND p.58).

1 Help the child into a semi-upright position supported by pillows. Incline his body towards the injured side. Cover any wounds to the chest wall using a sterile pad. Then seal with kitchen film. Secure pad on three sides with tape.

2 Place the arm on the injured side across your child's chest.

3 Support the raised arm in an ELEVATION SLING (see p.111). Keep him as comfortable as possible while you wait for the ambulance.

> **IF** *your child loses consciousness or develops breathing difficulties, assess his condition (see UNCONSCIOUS BABY, p.16; CHILD p.22). Be prepared to resuscitate.*

81

BROKEN ARM

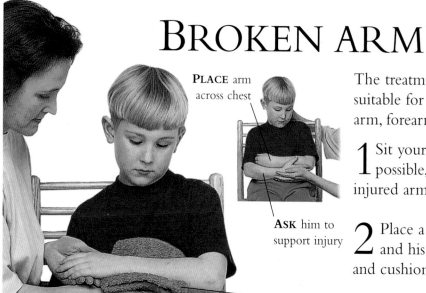

PLACE arm across chest

ASK him to support injury

PLACE padding around injury

The treatment described below is suitable for injuries to the upper arm, forearm, and wrist.

1 Sit your child down and, if possible, get him to support his injured arm in his hand.

2 Place a pad between his arm and his chest to immobilise and cushion the injured limb.

SUPPORT arm in a sling

TIE a broad-fold bandage around arm and chest

3 Put the injured limb in an ARM SLING (see p.110), secured with a REEF KNOT (see p.76).

4 For additional support, place a BROAD-FOLD BANDAGE over the sling and around your child's arm and chest (see p.76 and 80).

+ TAKE YOUR CHILD TO HOSPITAL

82

BROKEN ELBOW

Elbow injuries need special care and early treatment in hospital.
Recognising a broken elbow • *Pain increased by attempted movement* • *Stiffness* • *Swelling or bruising*

> **DO NOT** *attempt to straighten or bend the elbow.*

☎ CALL AN AMBULANCE

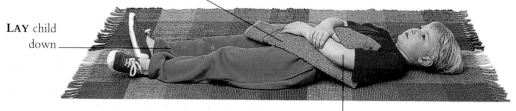

PUT soft padding between his arm and body

LAY child down

PLACE injured arm across his body

BROKEN HAND

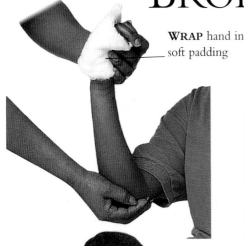

WRAP hand in soft padding

1 Wrap the injured hand in soft cotton wool padding. Raise your child's hand, supporting it to minimise swelling.

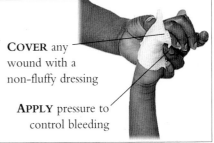

IF *there is a wound, control the bleeding by raising the hand and applying gentle pressure over a clean, non-fluffy pad.*

COVER any wound with a non-fluffy dressing

APPLY pressure to control bleeding

2 Place your child's arm in an ELEVATION SLING (see p.111) to reduce swelling and prevent movement of the injured hand.

SUPPORT hand and arm in elevation sling

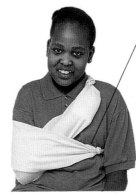

TIE broad-fold bandage around arm and body

3 Tie a BROAD-FOLD BANDAGE (see p.76 and 80) around the arm, securing it with a knot tied on the uninjured side.
✚ TAKE YOUR CHILD TO HOSPITAL

83

TRAPPED FINGERS

COOL injury by holding her fingers under running water

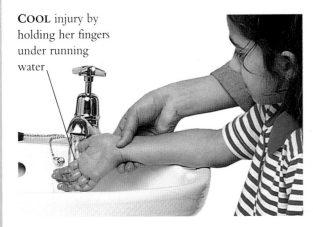

Hold the fingers under cold running water for a few minutes to relieve the pain and minimise swelling. If the fingers still hurt, apply a COLD COMPRESS (see p.84).

IF *after half an hour the fingers are still swollen and movement is impaired, they may be broken.*
✚ TAKE YOUR CHILD TO HOSPITAL

BRUISES AND SWELLINGS

After a fall or bump, bruising and swelling may develop rapidly. Resting, cooling, and elevating the injury will alleviate symptoms.

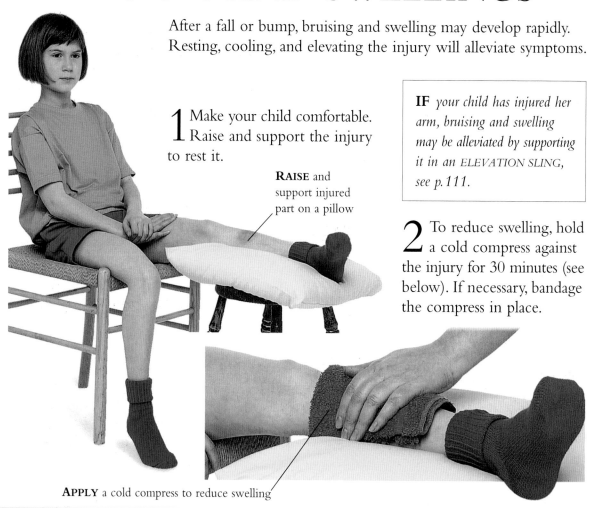

1 Make your child comfortable. Raise and support the injury to rest it.

RAISE and support injured part on a pillow

> **IF** *your child has injured her arm, bruising and swelling may be alleviated by supporting it in an ELEVATION SLING, see p.111.*

2 To reduce swelling, hold a cold compress against the injury for 30 minutes (see below). If necessary, bandage the compress in place.

84

APPLY a cold compress to reduce swelling

Making a cold compress

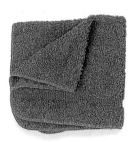

Cloth: wring it out in cold water and replace every ten minutes.

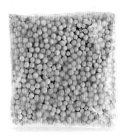

Bag of frozen peas: wrap in a light towel before placing it on the injury.

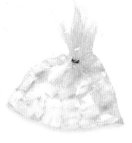

Ice: fill a plastic bag two-thirds full of ice and add a little salt to help the ice melt, then seal.

A cold compress minimises swelling and pain by reducing blood flow to the injured area. Leave a compress on the injury for about 30 minutes, changing it as necessary. If possible, the compress should be left uncovered, but if you need to secure it in place, use a gauze bandage or other open-weave material.

SPLINTER

1 Clean the area around the splinter with soap and warm water.

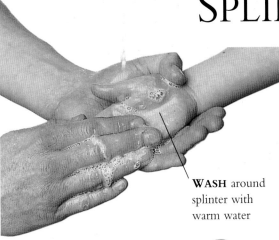

WASH around splinter with warm water

IF *your child is not inoculated against* TETANUS *(p.50),* ⓒ CALL A DOCTOR

DO NOT *poke at the area with a needle.*

2 Sterilise a pair of tweezers by passing them through a flame. Leave the tweezers to cool. Don't touch the ends or wipe off the soot.

STERILISE tweezers in a flame

85

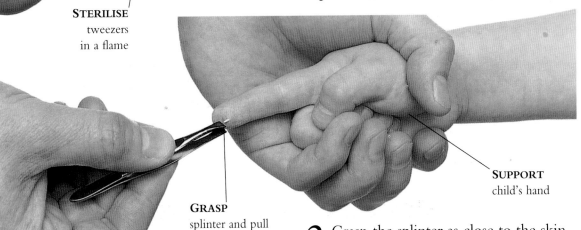

SUPPORT child's hand

GRASP splinter and pull straight out

3 Grasp the splinter as close to the skin as possible, and draw it back out at the angle it went in.

IF *the splinter doesn't come out easily, or if it breaks,* ⓒ CALL A DOCTOR

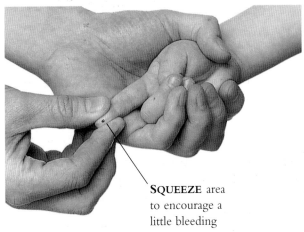

SQUEEZE area to encourage a little bleeding

4 Squeeze the wound to encourage a little bleeding that will flush out dirt. Wash the area again, pat it dry thoroughly, and cover with a plaster.

EYE

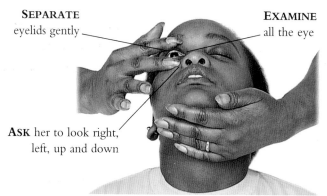

SEPARATE eyelids gently

EXAMINE all the eye

ASK her to look right, left, up and down

> **DO NOT** *touch, or attempt to remove, any foreign object that is sticking to, or embedded in, the eye, (see below).*

1 Sit your child down, facing the light. Separate the eyelids. Ask her to look right, left, up, and down. Examine all of the eye.

TRY to wash out foreign object

LIFT off foreign object with a damp swab

USE a bowl to catch water

2 If you can see the foreign object, wash it out using a jug of clean water. Tilt her head and aim for the inner corner so that water will wash over the eye. Or, use a damp swab or damp handkerchief to lift it off.

3 If an object is under the eyelid, you can ask an older child to clear it by lifting the upper eyelid over the lower. You will need to do this yourself for a younger child; wrap her in a towel first to stop her grabbing your arms.

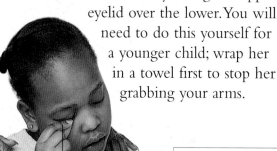

LIFT upper eyelid over lower lid

> **IF** *eye is still red or sore,*
> ✚ TAKE HER TO HOSPITAL

A foreign object that cannot be removed

Cover the eye with a sterile dressing. Reassure him.

✚ TAKE HIM TO HOSPITAL

COVER injured eye with a sterile dressing

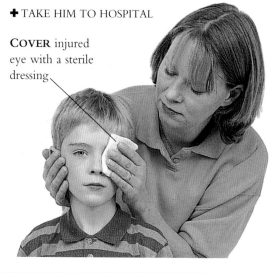

EAR

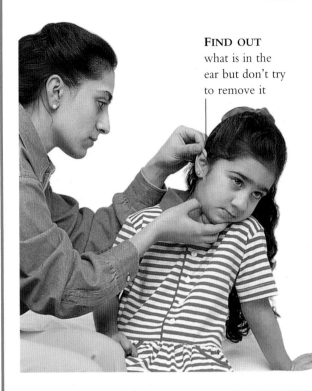

FIND OUT what is in the ear but don't try to remove it

Children often push things into their ears. A hard object may become stuck, causing pain and temporary deafness; it may damage the ear drum.

DO NOT *attempt to remove the object.*

Reassure your child and ask her what she put into her ear. Don't try to remove the object, even if you can see it.

✚ TAKE YOUR CHILD TO HOSPITAL

87

An insect in the ear

If an insect flies or crawls into the ear your child may be very alarmed. Sit her down and support her head with the affected ear uppermost. Gently flood the ear with tepid water so that the insect floats out.

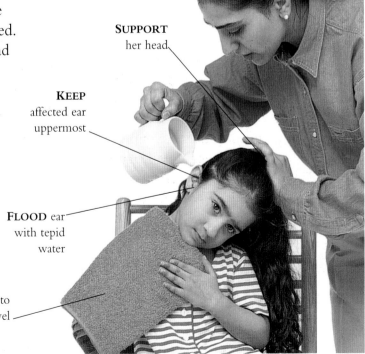

SUPPORT her head

KEEP affected ear uppermost

FLOOD ear with tepid water

ASK her to hold a towel

IF *you can't remove the insect,*
✚ TAKE YOUR CHILD TO HOSPITAL

NOSE

Recognising a foreign object in the nose
• *Difficult or noisy breathing through nose* • *Swelling of nose* • *Smelly or blood-stained discharge indicates object has been present for a while*

Calm and reassure your child and tell him to breathe through his mouth.

> **DO NOT** *attempt to remove the object.*
> ✚ TAKE YOUR CHILD TO HOSPITAL

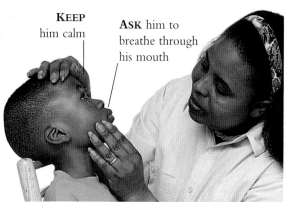

KEEP him calm

ASK him to breathe through his mouth

SWALLOWED OBJECT

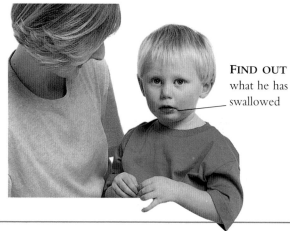

FIND OUT what he has swallowed

Find out what your child has swallowed. If the object is small and smooth like a pebble or a coin, there is little danger.

✆ CALL A DOCTOR

> **IF** *the object is sharp or large, don't give your child anything to eat or drink.*
> ✚ TAKE YOUR CHILD TO HOSPITAL

INHALED FOREIGN OBJECT

Small, smooth objects can slip into the air passages. Peanuts are a danger in young children as they can be inhaled into the lungs.

Your child will cough violently and this may expel the object. If he continues to choke, see CHOKING BABY p.36; CHILD p.38.

✆ CALL A DOCTOR OR
✚ TAKE HIM TO HOSPITAL

GIVE up to five abdominal thrusts if he continues to choke after back slaps and chest thrusts

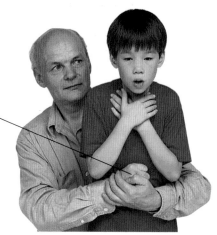

88

ANIMAL BITE
Superficial bite

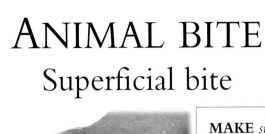

WASH wound with soap and warm, running water

MAKE *sure he is protected against tetanus infection (see p.50).*

1 Wash the wound thoroughly, using soap and warm water. Rinse the wound under running water for at least five minutes to wash away any dirt.

2 Gently, but thoroughly, pat the wound dry with a clean pad or tissue. Cover it with a plaster or a small sterile dressing.

DRY wound and cover with a plaster

C CALL A DOCTOR

Serious bite

89

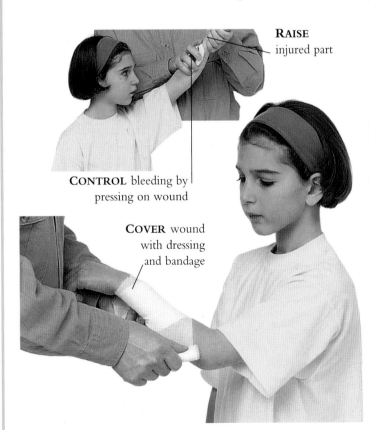

RAISE injured part

CONTROL bleeding by pressing on wound

COVER wound with dressing and bandage

1 Apply direct pressure over the wound, preferably over a clean dressing or pad. Lift and support the injured part above the level of your child's heart.

IF *the bleeding is severe, see* BLEEDING, *p.46.*

2 Cover the wound with a sterile dressing or pad and bandage firmly in place.

+ TAKE YOUR CHILD TO HOSPITAL

IF *your child is bitten by an animal while you are abroad, or if the bite comes from an animal smuggled into the UK, you must take your child to hospital for anti-rabies injections.*

INSECT STING

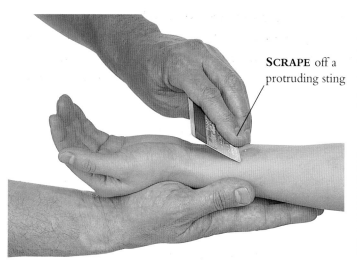

SCRAPE off a protruding sting

1 If the sting is still in the skin, brush or scrape it off sideways. Do not try to remove it with tweezers as you will inject more poison into your child.

IF *your child collapses, she may be allergic to the sting. Follow the treatment for ANAPHYLACTIC SHOCK, opposite.*

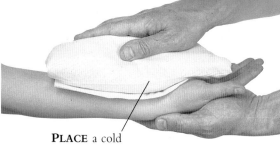

PLACE a cold compress over area

2 Cool the area with a COLD COMPRESS (see p.84) to minimise the pain and swelling. Leave the compress in place for about ten minutes, until the pain is relieved. Rest the injured part.

Sting in mouth

To reduce swelling, give your child an ice cube to suck or cold water to drink.

C CALL A DOCTOR

IF her breathing becomes difficult, ☎ CALL AN AMBULANCE

NETTLE RASH

To relieve the itching, dab the rash with cotton wool soaked in calamine lotion. Alternatively, place a COLD COMPRESS (see p.84) over the rash until the pain is relieved, about ten minutes. If the rash is extensive,

C CALL A DOCTOR

SOOTHE rash by dabbing with calamine lotion

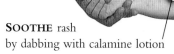

ANAPHYLACTIC SHOCK

This is a severe allergic reaction that may develop within a few minutes following the injection of a particular drug, the sting of an insect or marine creature, or the ingestion of a particular food.

The reaction causes constriction of the air passages. Swelling of the face and neck increases the risk of suffocation.

Recognising anaphylactic shock
• *Anxiety* • *Red, blotchy skin* • *Swelling of the face and neck* • *Puffiness around the eyes*
• *Wheezing* • *Difficult breathing* • *Rapid pulse*

☎ CALL AN AMBULANCE

> **IF** *your child loses consciousness, assess his condition (see* UNCONSCIOUS BABY *p.16;* CHILD *p.22). If breathing, place him in the* RECOVERY POSITION. *Be prepared to resuscitate.*

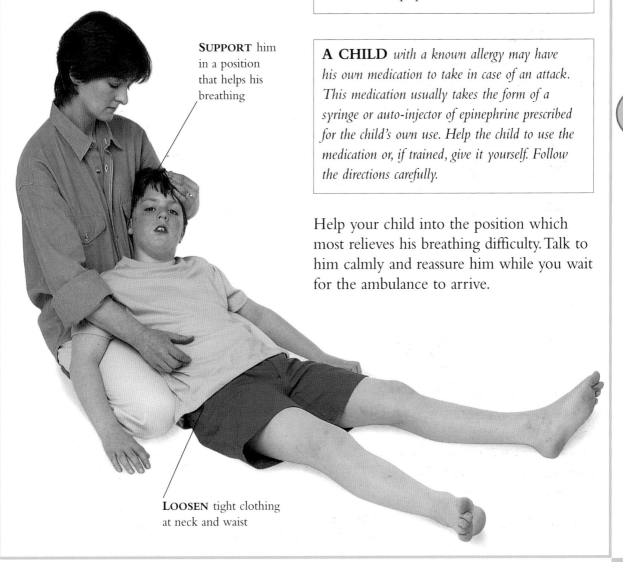

SUPPORT him in a position that helps his breathing

LOOSEN tight clothing at neck and waist

> **A CHILD** *with a known allergy may have his own medication to take in case of an attack. This medication usually takes the form of a syringe or auto-injector of epinephrine prescribed for the child's own use. Help the child to use the medication or, if trained, give it yourself. Follow the directions carefully.*

Help your child into the position which most relieves his breathing difficulty. Talk to him calmly and reassure him while you wait for the ambulance to arrive.

91

MARINE STINGS
Jellyfish sting

Jellyfish venom is contained in stinging cells that stick to a child's skin. The sting is painful, but not usually serious. A similar reaction is produced by sea anemones and corals.

IF *your child develops a severe allergic reaction, see ANAPHYLACTIC SHOCK p.91.* ☎ CALL AN AMBULANCE

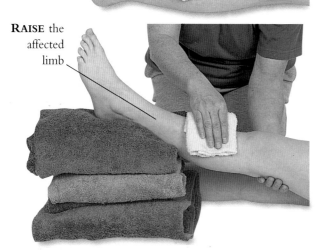

COOL the affected area

1 Apply a cold compress against the skin for about ten minutes.

RAISE the affected limb

2 If possible, raise the affected part to reduce swelling.

IF *the skin is very red and painful,* ✚ TAKE YOUR CHILD TO HOSPITAL

92

Weever fish sting

When trodden on, the spines from weever fish can puncture the skin, causing painful swelling and soreness. The spines may break off and become embedded in the foot.

Immerse the injury in water as hot as your child can bear for at least 30 minutes. Top up as the water cools but be careful not to scald her.

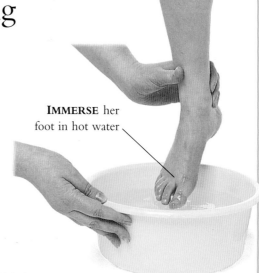

IMMERSE her foot in hot water

IF *any spines remain, or the foot starts to swell,* ✚ TAKE YOUR CHILD TO HOSPITAL

SNAKE BITE

Recognising a snake bite • *A pair of puncture marks* • *Severe pain, redness, and swelling around bite* • *Vomiting* • *Disturbed vision* • *Breathing difficulties* • *Increased salivation and sweating*

IF *your child develops* ANAPHYLACTIC SHOCK, *see p.91.* **IF** *he loses consciousness, see* UNCONSCIOUS BABY *p.16;* CHILD *p.22. Be prepared to resuscitate. If breathing, place him in the* RECOVERY POSITION.

DO NOT *let your child walk.*
DO NOT *apply a tourniquet, cut out the wound, or try to suck out the venom.*
An accurate description of the snake will help doctors treat the injury.

1 Help your child to lie down. Keep the heart above the level of the bite area to contain the poison.

2 Gently wash the wound and pat dry with clean swabs.

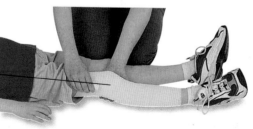

CLEAN and dry the wound

93

RAISE the heart above the level of the bite

APPLY a roller bandage above the wound

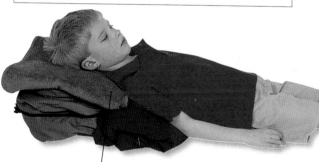

3 Lightly compress the limb above the wound with a roller bandage. If the hand or foot begins to feel numb or cold, loosen the bandages slightly.

4 Immobilize the limb with folded triangular bandages and padding.

5 Reassure him. Keep him still to stop the venom spreading through his body.

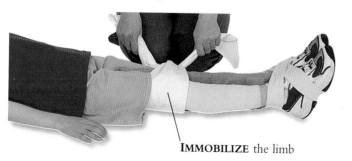

IMMOBILIZE the limb

☎ CALL AN AMBULANCE

HYPOTHERMIA

Hypothermia occurs when the body temperature falls. Deep hypothermia, where the body temperature has fallen to a very low level, is extremely serious. An older child is most likely to develop hypothermia after over-exertion outside in poor weather conditions, or after falling into very cold water. For babies, see opposite.

GIVE her a warm bath

Recognising hypothermia
- *Shivering* • *Cold, pale, dry skin*
- *Listlessness or confusion* • *Failing consciousness* • *Slow, shallow breathing*
- *Weakening pulse*

1 Give your child a warm bath, if she is able to climb in herself. When her skin colour has returned to normal, help her out, dry her quickly, and wrap her in warm towels or blankets.

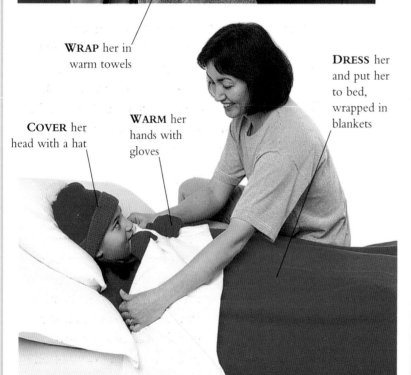

WRAP her in warm towels

DRESS her and put her to bed, wrapped in blankets

COVER her head with a hat

WARM her hands with gloves

2 Dress your child with warm clothes and put her to bed, covered with plenty of blankets. Cover her head with a hat and make sure that the room is warm. Stay with her.

✆ CALL A DOCTOR

> **DO NOT** *put a source of direct heat, such as a hot-water bottle, next to the child's skin. The child must warm up gradually.*

94

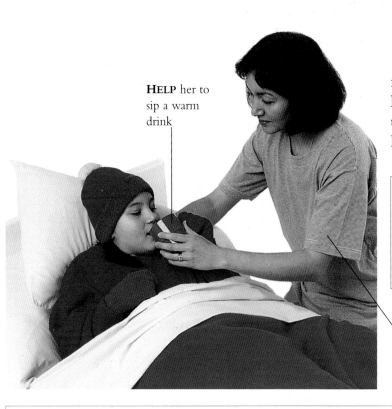

HELP her to sip a warm drink

3 Give your child a warm drink and some high-energy foods, such as chocolate. Do not leave her alone until you are sure that her colour and temperature have returned to normal.

> IF *your child loses consciousness, assess her condition (see* UNCONSCIOUS BABY *p.16;* CHILD *p.22). Be prepared to resuscitate.*
> ☎ CALL AN AMBULANCE

STAY with her until colour and temperature have returned to normal

Hypothermia in babies

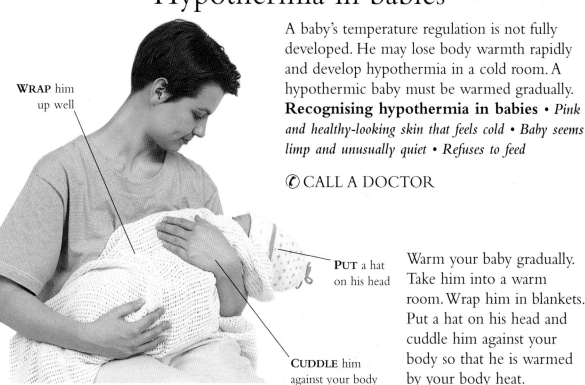

WRAP him up well

A baby's temperature regulation is not fully developed. He may lose body warmth rapidly and develop hypothermia in a cold room. A hypothermic baby must be warmed gradually.
Recognising hypothermia in babies • *Pink and healthy-looking skin that feels cold* • *Baby seems limp and unusually quiet* • *Refuses to feed*

© CALL A DOCTOR

PUT a hat on his head

Warm your baby gradually. Take him into a warm room. Wrap him in blankets. Put a hat on his head and cuddle him against your body so that he is warmed by your body heat.

CUDDLE him against your body

FROSTBITE

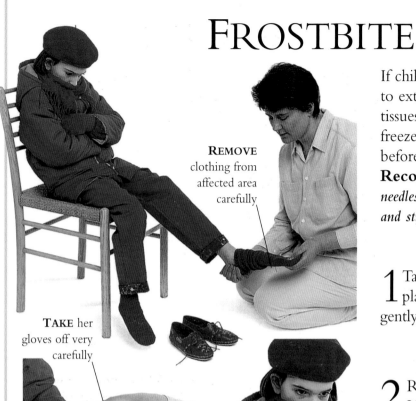

REMOVE clothing from affected area carefully

If children are accidentally exposed to extreme weather conditions, the tissues of the fingers and toes may freeze. Get your child to shelter before you start treatment.

Recognising frostbite • *Pins and needles* • *Numbing* • *Skin feeling hard and stiff, turning white, and waxy*

1 Take your child into a warm place. Sit her down then very gently remove her socks and shoes.

TAKE her gloves off very carefully

2 Remove gloves and any rings. Undo her coat. Tell her to warm her hands under her armpits.

WARM hands with her own body heat, under armpits

3 When the feet or toes are frozen, to reduce swelling and provide warmth, raise your child's feet and warm her toes under your own armpits.

USE your body heat to thaw feet

> **DO NOT** *warm by rubbing or with direct heat, such as hot-water bottles.* **NEVER** *burst blisters.*

4 If the skin is broken or the colour does not return rapidly, apply a soft gauze dressing and bandage it lightly in place.
✚ TAKE YOUR CHILD TO HOSPITAL

COVER with light dressing and bandage if colour does not return

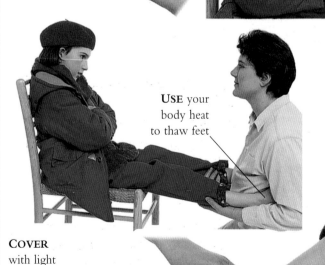

96

HEAT EXHAUSTION

This condition may develop in hot, humid weather and is caused by dehydration. Children who are unwell, particularly with diarrhoea and vomiting, and those not used to playing in the heat are most at risk.

Recognising heat exhaustion • *Headache and dizziness* • *Nausea* • *Sweating* • *Pale, clammy skin* • *Cramps* • *Rapid, weakening pulse*

1 Take your child into the shade or into a cool room. Help him to lie down.

LAY child down in cool room

PUT folded towel or cushion under his head

2 Raise and support your child's legs on some pillows. This improves blood supply to the brain. Encourage him to rest.

97

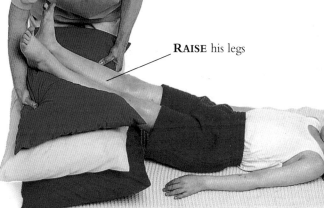

RAISE his legs

3 Help your child to sit up and sip as much cool, salty water (a solution of 5ml/1 teaspoon of salt per litre of fluid) or juice as he can manage. This replaces salt lost from the body.

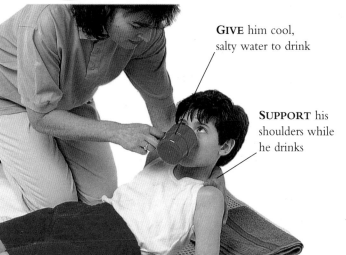

GIVE him cool, salty water to drink

SUPPORT his shoulders while he drinks

> **IF** *he loses consciousness, assess his condition (see* UNCONSCIOUS BABY *p16;* CHILD, *p.22). Be prepared to resuscitate. If breathing, place him in the* RECOVERY POSITION.
> ☎ CALL AN AMBULANCE

HEATSTROKE

If the body becomes severely overheated in hot surroundings, heatstroke may occur.

Recognising heatstroke

- *Sudden onset of headache*
- *Confusion* • *Hot, flushed, dry skin* • *Rapid deterioration in level of response* • *A full, bounding pulse* • *Temperature above 40°C (104°F)*

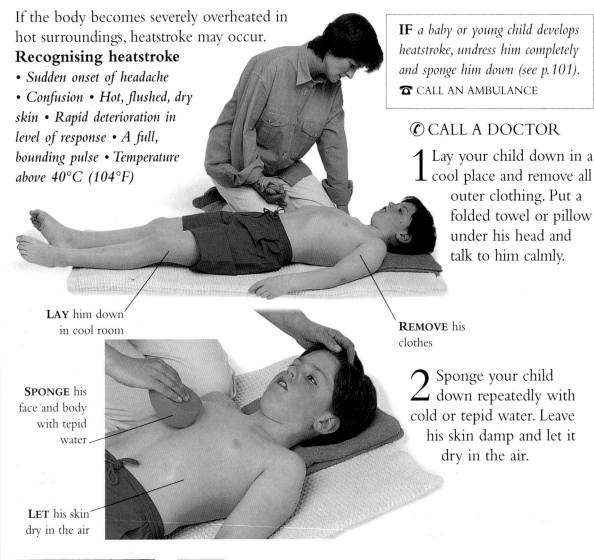

LAY him down in cool room

REMOVE his clothes

SPONGE his face and body with tepid water

LET his skin dry in the air

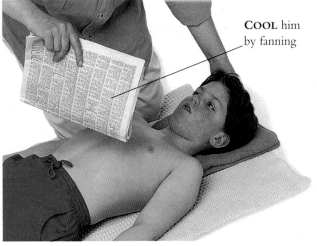

COOL him by fanning

IF *a baby or young child develops heatstroke, undress him completely and sponge him down (see p.101).*
☎ CALL AN AMBULANCE

ⓒ CALL A DOCTOR

1 Lay your child down in a cool place and remove all outer clothing. Put a folded towel or pillow under his head and talk to him calmly.

2 Sponge your child down repeatedly with cold or tepid water. Leave his skin damp and let it dry in the air.

3 Fan your child by hand or with an electric fan to bring his temperature down.

IF *he loses consciousness, assess his condition (see UNCONSCIOUS BABY p16; CHILD, p.22). Be prepared to resuscitate. If breathing, place him in the RECOVERY POSITION.*
☎ CALL AN AMBULANCE

98

SUNBURN

Sunburn is red, itchy, and tender. Babies and young children are particularly vulnerable and should wear a hat and protective cream or clothing in the sun.

IF *there is blistering,*
ⓒ CALL A DOCTOR

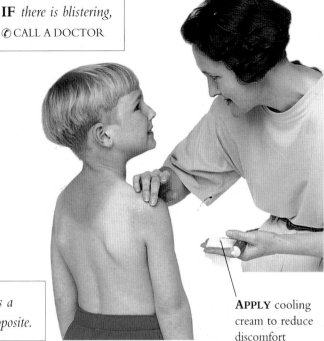

TAKE him into shade

GIVE him cold water to sip

1 Move your child into the shade or into a cool room and give him a cold drink.

2 Apply calamine cream or a special after-sun cream to soothe the skin.

IF *your child is restless, flushed, dizzy, or has a temperature or headache, see HEATSTROKE, opposite.*

APPLY cooling cream to reduce discomfort

99

HEAT RASH

Recognising heat rash • *A prickly, red rash particularly around the sweat glands on the chest and back and under the arms*

Sit your child down in a cool room and undress her. Sponge her down with cool water. Pat her almost dry with a soft towel, leaving the skin slightly damp. Apply calamine cream.

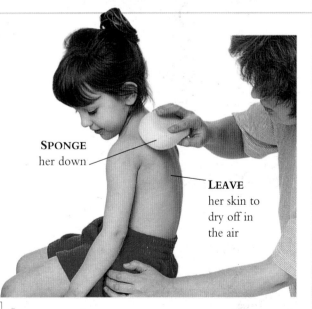

SPONGE her down

LEAVE her skin to dry off in the air

IF *your baby develops heat rash, remove some of her clothes to cool her, or bathe her in tepid water. Dry her gently, leaving her skin slightly damp.*

IF *the rash has not faded after 12 hours, or if her temperature is raised,* ⓒ CALL A DOCTOR

FEVER

A body temperature that is above the normal level of 37°C (98.6°F) indicates fever. An infection is the usual cause. If your child also has a bad headache, you should study the information on MENINGITIS (see opposite). A moderate fever is not harmful, but a temperature of above 40°C (104°F) can be dangerous, particularly in babies and very young children.

Recognising a fever • *Raised temperature* • *A very pale face and a chilled feeling, with goose pimples* • *Shivering, with chattering teeth* As the fever advances • *Hot, flushed skin* • *General achiness* • *Sweating* • *Headache*

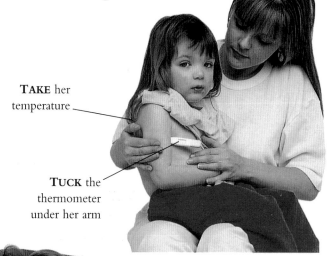

TAKE her temperature

TUCK the thermometer under her arm

1 Lift your child's arm and tuck the pointed end of the thermometer into her armpit. Fold her arm over her chest and leave the thermometer in place for the recommended time. A digital thermometer is the easiest to use.

LAY her down in bed or on the sofa

2 Make your child comfortable on a bed or sofa, but do not cover her. To help bring down her temperature, make sure she has plenty of water or diluted fruit juice to drink.

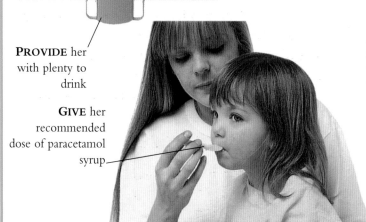

PROVIDE her with plenty to drink

GIVE her recommended dose of paracetamol syrup

3 You can give your child the recommended dose of paracetamol syrup to help reduce her temperature. If your child is very hot, sponge her down as well, (see opposite).

> **IF** *your baby is under three months old, she should not be given paracetamol syrup, unless you are advised to do so by your doctor.*

Cooling babies and young children

In babies and children under four years of age, there is some risk of FEBRILE SEIZURES (see p.32). If your child's temperature rises above 40°C (104°F),

© CALL A DOCTOR

UNDRESS him

COOL him by sponging with tepid water

Babies

Undress your baby down to his nappy and cool him by lightly sponging his body with tepid water. Try to keep him calm.

Young children

Undress your child and cool her by sponging her with tepid water. Continue for up to 30 minutes. Take her temperature again.

LET his skin dry in the air

FEVER *can also be caused by too much sun, see HEATSTROKE, p.98.*

101

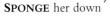
SPONGE her down

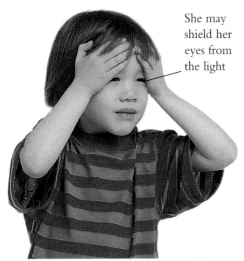
LET her skin dry in the air

Meningitis

She may shield her eyes from the light

This is a serious condition involving the tissues that surround the brain. It is frequently life-threatening and urgent treatment is essential.

Recognising meningitis Your child may develop
• *Fever* • *Vomiting* • *Headache* • *Neck pain or stiffness* • *Seizures* • *A red or purple rash that does not fade when pressure is applied* • *Pain in the eyes caused by light*

© CALL A DOCTOR URGENTLY

IF *there is any delay in help arriving,*
✚ TAKE YOUR CHILD TO HOSPITAL OR
☎ CALL AN AMBULANCE

VOMITING

HOLD a bowl
for her

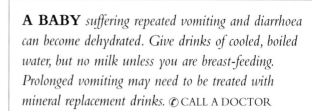

> **A BABY** *suffering repeated vomiting and diarrhoea can become dehydrated. Give drinks of cooled, boiled water, but no milk unless you are breast-feeding. Prolonged vomiting may need to be treated with mineral replacement drinks.* ℭ CALL A DOCTOR

1 Hold your child over a bowl or basin. Support her upper body with your free hand while she is being sick. Reassure her.

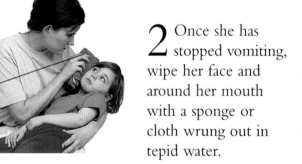

2 Once she has stopped vomiting, wipe her face and around her mouth with a sponge or cloth wrung out in tepid water.

SPONGE her face gently

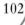

GIVE her water to drink

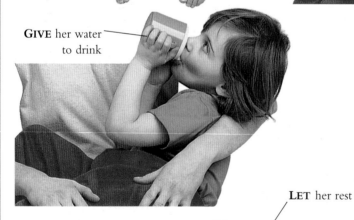

3 Give her drinks of water to replace any fluid loss and to remove the unpleasant taste. Encourage her to sip each drink slowly.

LET her rest

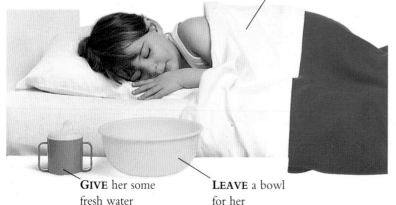

4 Let her rest quietly, in bed if she wants to. Make sure the bowl is still at hand for further sickness attacks, and provide a fresh drink of water.

GIVE her some
fresh water

LEAVE a bowl
for her

STOMACHACHE

PROP her up against cushions or pillows

1 Make your child comfortable on a sofa or bed. If she is having difficulty breathing, help her to lie back against cushions or pillows. She may want to be sick so leave a container nearby.

> **IF** *the pain is severe, or does not subside after 30 minutes,*
> ℭ CALL A DOCTOR

2 Warmth may help to relieve the pain. Fill a hot-water bottle – it must be covered – and give it to your child to hold against her stomach. Avoid giving her anything to eat.

PROVIDE a bowl if she feels sick

GIVE her a covered hot-water bottle to hold against her stomach

103

Appendicitis

Inflammation of the appendix is rare under the age of two but may affect older, especially teenage, children.

Recognising appendicitis • *Waves of pain in the middle of the abdomen* • *Acute pain settling in the right lower abdomen* • *Raised temperature* • *Loss of appetite* • *Nausea* • *Vomiting* • *Diarrhoea*

> **APPENDICITIS** *must be treated promptly. Help your child to lie down on a sofa or bed. Do not give him anything to eat or drink.*
> ℭ CALL A DOCTOR

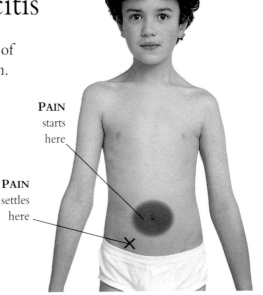

PAIN starts here

PAIN settles here

EARACHE

1 Make your child comfortable. Sit her up supported by pillows or cushions if lying flat makes the earache worse. Give her the recommended dose of paracetamol syrup.

GIVE her recommended dose of paracetamol syrup

PROP her up

2 Applying heat may help to soothe the pain. Prepare a covered hot-water bottle and tell your child to lie down with her painful ear against it.

PROVIDE a covered hot-water bottle to place against her ear

IF *pain does not begin to subside, or if there is a discharge from the ear, fever, or hearing loss,* ℂ CALL A DOCTOR

104

Pressure-change earache

This may happen on plane journeys, particularly when taking off or landing, or when travelling through tunnels. To make the ears "pop" so that the pressure is relieved, your child should close her mouth, hold her nose and blow down it. Sucking a sweet may also help.

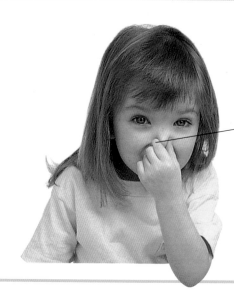

TELL her to pinch her nose, close her mouth, and "blow" her nose

TOOTHACHE

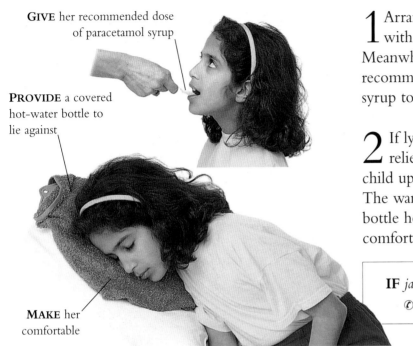

GIVE her recommended dose of paracetamol syrup

PROVIDE a covered hot-water bottle to lie against

MAKE her comfortable

1 Arrange an early appointment with your child's dentist. Meanwhile, give her the recommended dose of paracetamol syrup to relieve the pain.

2 If lying down does not help to relieve the pain, prop your child up with pillows or cushions. The warmth of a covered hot-water bottle held against the cheek may comfort her.

> **IF** *jaw is swollen and pain is severe,*
> ℭ CALL A DOCTOR

105

CRAMP

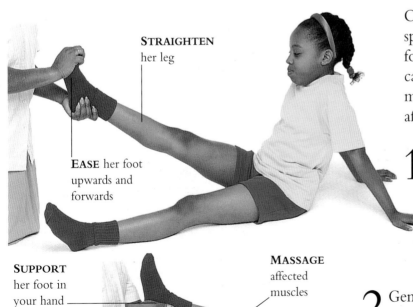

STRAIGHTEN her leg

EASE her foot upwards and forwards

SUPPORT her foot in your hand

MASSAGE affected muscles

Cramp is a painful muscle spasm that often affects the foot and calf muscles. You can relieve the pain by massaging and stretching the affected muscles.

1 Help your child to sit down then raise her leg and straighten her knee. Ease her toes upwards to flex the foot.

2 Gently but firmly knead the affected muscle with your fingertips until the spasm has passed completely.

A well-stocked first aid kit

1 small roller bandage
1 large roller bandage
1 small conforming bandage
1 large conforming bandage
Scissors
Calamine cream
Pack of gauze swabs
2 triangular bandages
Hypoallergenic tape
2 sterile pads
Waterproof plasters
1 finger bandage and applicator
Tweezers
1 sterile dressing with bandage

FIRST AID KIT

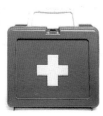

Keep first aid kits in your car and in your home. You can buy ready-made-up standard kits. You may want to add extra dressings and bandages, and disposable gloves. Make sure your first aid box is readily accessible and easy to identify, and check the contents regularly. Don't keep medicines in the first aid box; they should be locked in a medicine cabinet. A well-stocked kit might contain the articles shown below.

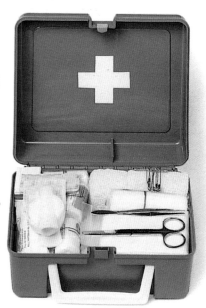

106

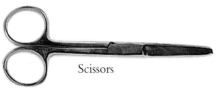

Scissors

Dressings

Plasters (adhesive dressings) are used for minor wounds. Keep several different sizes and shapes. Keep a selection of larger sterile dressings for more serious wounds.

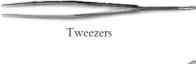

Tweezers

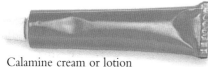

Calamine cream or lotion

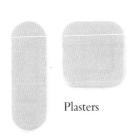

Plasters

Gauze swabs

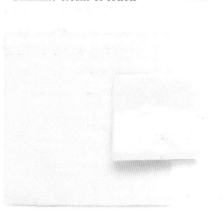

Sterile non-adhesive pad

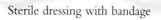

Sterile dressing with bandage

Bandages

Keep a variety of bandages to secure dressings and support injured joints. Conforming bandages shape themselves to the contours of the body and so are easy to use. Triangular bandages can be used as slings and for broad- and narrow-fold bandages.

Hypoallergenic tape for securing dressings

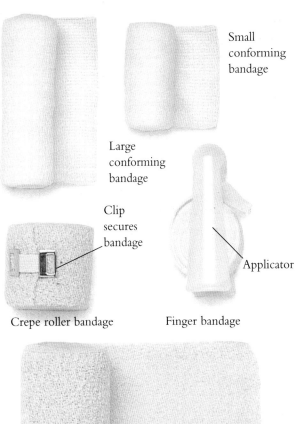

Small conforming bandage

Large conforming bandage

Clip secures bandage

Applicator

Crepe roller bandage

Finger bandage

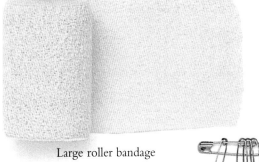

Large roller bandage

Safety pins

Folded triangular bandage

Other useful items

A variety of household items are invaluable for first aid emergencies. If you don't have exactly the right materials, you can improvise successfully. Keep the following articles to hand.

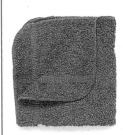

Flannel
Use a flannel soaked in water to make a cold compress or to sponge a child with a fever.

Sheet and pillow case
A clean cotton sheet or pillowcase makes an excellent loose protective covering for burns.

Kitchen film
Plastic kitchen film can be used to dress burns and seal chest wounds.

Plastic bags
A clean plastic bag can be put over a burned foot or hand and lightly secured with bandages or tape.

107

DRESSINGS

Covering a wound with a dressing will help prevent infection and help the blood-clotting process. Dressings should not be fluffy and need to be large enough to cover the wound and the surrounding area. Always wash your hands before you apply dressings and wear disposable gloves if you have them. If blood soaks through a dressing, place another on top. Make sure any bandages are not too tight (see opposite).

Plaster

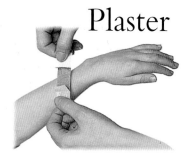

Remove wrapping and, holding the pad over the wound, peel back the protective strips. Press the ends and edges down.

Sterile pad

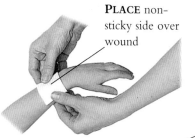

PLACE non-sticky side over wound

BANDAGE the pad in place

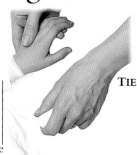

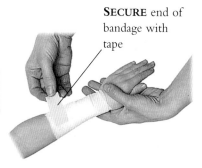

SECURE end of bandage with tape

1 Place the pad shiny side down directly over the child's wound.

2 Secure the pad with a bandage, working from below the injury up the limb.

3 Secure the end of the bandage with hypoallergenic tape.

Sterile dressing with bandage

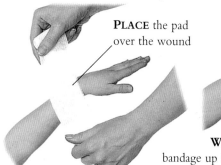

PLACE the pad over the wound

WIND the bandage up the limb

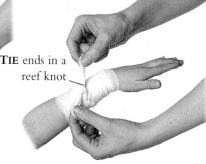

TIE ends in a reef knot

1 Hold the bandage either side of the dressing, and place the pad over the wound.

2 Leaving the short end hanging, wind the other end around the limb until the dressing is covered.

3 Tie the two ends of the bandage in a REEF KNOT (see p.76), over the pad.

108

BANDAGING

Use bandages to secure dressings, to help control bleeding, and to support injuries. Roller bandages can be used for any part of the body; conforming bandages are especially useful for bandaging joints or heads as they mould themselves to the shape of the body.

DO NOT *apply a bandage too tightly – it will impair the circulation. To check, press on your child's nail or a patch of skin, then release pressure. The colour should return rapidly. If it does not, loosen the bandages.*

Roller bandage

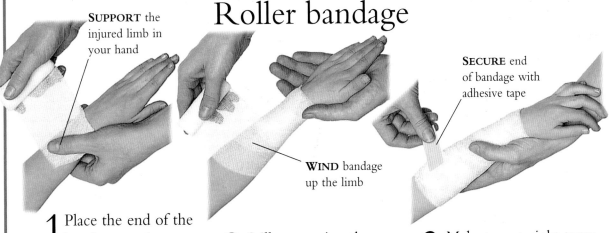

SUPPORT the injured limb in your hand

WIND bandage up the limb

SECURE end of bandage with adhesive tape

1 Place the end of the bandage on the arm below the injury and hold the bandage roll in your other hand.

2 Still supporting the injury, wind the bandage around the arm, winding up the limb.

3 Make two straight turns to finish. Secure the end with tape. Check your child's circulation (see above).

Hand bandage

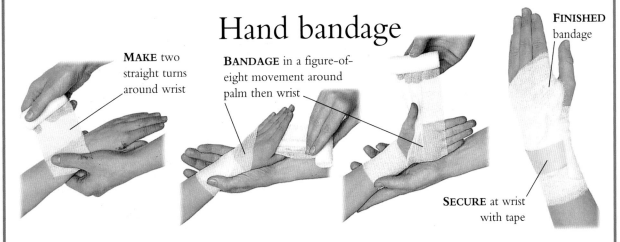

MAKE two straight turns around wrist

BANDAGE in a figure-of-eight movement around palm then wrist

FINISHED bandage

SECURE at wrist with tape

1 Supporting the injury, hold the end of the bandage on the wrist and make two straight turns.

2 Take the bandage across the back of the hand to the base of the little finger, then around the palm, and up between the thumb and forefinger, and across the back of the hand to the wrist. Repeat the "figure-of-eight" until the hand is covered.

109

TRIANGULAR BANDAGES

These are sold singly in sterile packs or can be made from a square of strong fabric folded diagonally in half. Triangular bandages are used for BROAD-FOLD and NARROW-FOLD BANDAGES (see p.76) or slings. Arm slings support injured arms or wrists, or take weight off an injured shoulder. Elevation slings are used for arm and upper body injuries where bleeding, pain, or swelling need to be reduced. (For REEF KNOT see p.76.)

Arm sling

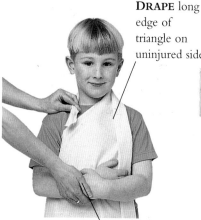

DRAPE long edge of triangle on uninjured side

SUPPORT arm

1 Place the bandage between your child's arm and chest, easing one end up around the back of his neck on the injured side.

TIE a reef knot at shoulder

2 Take the lower end of the bandage up over your child's forearm to the end at the shoulder and tie a REEF KNOT (see p.76) just below the shoulder.

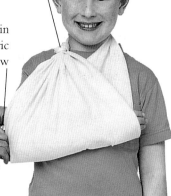

MAKE the reef knot comfortable

BRING lower end up over forearm

TUCK in surplus fabric at elbow

3 Fold in the surplus fabric at the corner near the elbow and pin it to the bandage.

Improvised slings

If your child injures her shoulder, arm, or hand out of doors, you can improvise a sling to support the injury until she receives further treatment.

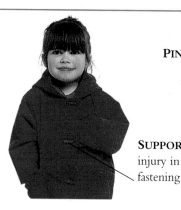

SUPPORT injury in coat fastening

Undo a coat button and tuck the hand of the injured arm inside the fastening.

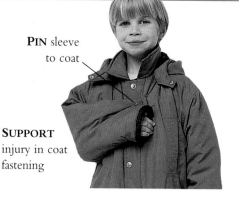

PIN sleeve to coat

Alternatively, pin your child's sleeve up on the opposite side of his chest.

110

Elevation sling

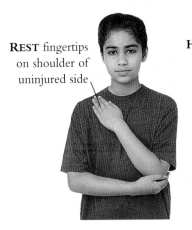

REST fingertips on shoulder of uninjured side

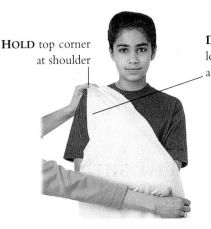

HOLD top corner at shoulder

DRAPE long edge across body

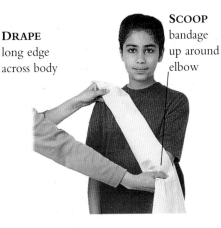

SCOOP bandage up around elbow

1 Bring the arm on the injured side across your child's chest. Ask her to support her elbow.

2 Lay the bandage over your child's arm, with the long edge hanging on the uninjured side. Hold the top corner at the shoulder.

3 Fold long edge of bandage in under injured arm.

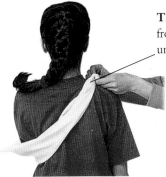

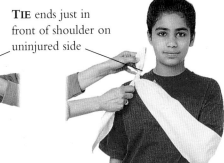

TIE ends just in front of shoulder on uninjured side

4 Bring the other end up around her back, holding the elbow securely in the fabric. Tie a REEF KNOT (p.76) just below the shoulder and tuck the ends in.

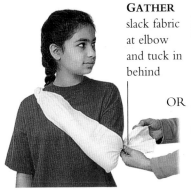

GATHER slack fabric at elbow and tuck in behind

OR

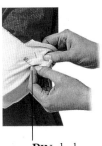

PIN slack fabric to front of sling

5 Secure the bandage by twisting the excess fabric and tucking it in at the elbow. Pin in place.

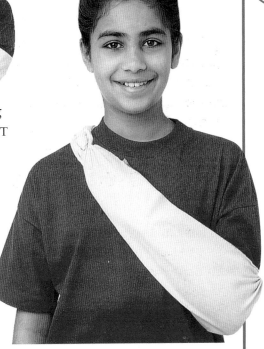

Finished sling raises, immobilizes, and supports the injury.

SAFETY IN THE HOME

Most accidents occur at home and over half involve children under the age of five. Many accidents are preventable if you:

- Alter the layout and position of objects and furniture at home.
- Make sure that all windows are closed or inaccessible.
- Never confuse containers by putting a dangerous substance, such as bleach, in a bottle that used to contain a harmless drink.
- Never tell your child that medicines and pills are special sweeties.
- Check for potential hazards when visiting friends or relatives and ask if you can move sharp or breakable objects.
- Teach your child basic safety rules.

ELECTRICITY

Protect your child from electric shock (see p.12).

- Cover sockets: put heavy furniture in front of them, or fit plastic covers.
- Put only one or two plugs into each socket – overloading can start a fire.
- Wire plugs safely – follow instructions and check that you have the right fuse.
- Check that old flexes are not worn – a child may try to chew protuding wires.
- Tidy up trailing wires.
- Unplug electrical appliances at night, particularly the television.
- Fit an RCD (residual current device).

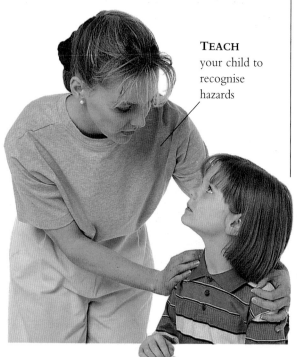

TEACH your child to recognise hazards

GAS

Find out where your gas tap is in case there is a leak. If you smell gas:

- Don't turn the lights on or off or use any electric switches – there might be a spark, which could cause an explosion.
- Don't light matches or cigarettes.
- Turn off the gas.
- Open the windows.
- Call the gas company.

FIRE

If fire breaks out at home, it could be a matter of minutes before smoke overcomes you.

Fit at least one smoke detector per floor
If your house is on one level, fit a detector between the sitting room and the bedrooms. If your house is on two or more levels, fit one detector at the foot of the stairs and another outside the bedrooms upstairs.

Have an escape plan (see p. 11). Make sure the whole family knows what to do if there is a fire.

Practise a fire drill with your children

- Shout "fire" • Set off the smoke detector • Tell everyone to drop to the floor and crawl to the exit from the room • Shut the door behind you • Don't go back for pets or treasured possessions.

KEEP *emergency numbers by the telephone, and make sure the babysitter knows where they are.*

HALL AND STAIRS

The staircase is not a safe place for your child to play (see below).

- Make sure that toys are not left there for you to trip over.
- Put a light in your hall or on the landing in case your child gets up at night. Use a low watt bulb; never cover a lamp with a cloth as the cloth can easily catch fire.
- Don't let your child play on the landings or stairs of a communal area in flats as the banisters may have large gaps between them.

FRONT DOOR

- Don't leave your front door open.
- Don't let your child answer the door to callers.
- Put the door catch out of reach of small children. If your toddler can reach the catch, fix an additional bolt higher up the door and always keep the door bolted.
- Stick plastic safety film over glass doors. This stops the glass from splintering if it gets broken. Better still, fit toughened or laminated glass.
- Put stickers over the glass to make it more noticeable for young children.

FLOOR

Tiled, polished, or hessian-covered floors can be very slippery for toddlers and running children.

- Put non-slip webbing under rugs.
- Keep hall floors free of toys and clutter.
- Check fitted carpets regularly for holes or loose carpet that might catch a toddler's foot.

STAIRS

A child is not co-ordinated enough to be able to walk downstairs safely until he is at least three years old.

- Fit stair gates at the foot and top of the stairs. Vertical posts on stair gates should be no more than 6.5cm (2½in) apart. A young child can get through a larger gap and fall, or get his head stuck. Always open the gate when you are going upstairs or downstairs. Do not climb over it: your children will learn from you.
- Check your banisters for safety. Make sure the handrail is sturdy and check regularly for loose posts. Posts should be no more than 10cm (4in) apart. Do not let your child use the rails as a climbing frame.
- Check the stair carpet. Loose carpet or worn steps can be a hazard.

113

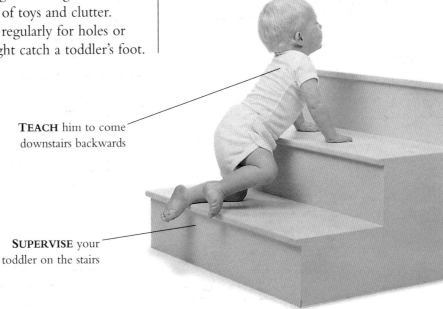

TEACH him to come downstairs backwards

SUPERVISE your toddler on the stairs

KITCHEN

The kitchen may be the busiest part of your house, where you spend a lot of time with your children. Constant bustle and cooking activities make it a potentially hazardous area.

DOOR
- Cover any glass panels with safety film to stop them shattering or splintering should your toddler run into the door.
- Put some colourful stickers on the glass to alert your child.

FLOOR
- Don't let your child play on the area of floor between you and the work surface or where you could trip over him.
- Avoid bumps and falls by wiping up spills immediately.
- Remove pet food bowls after use and keep that part of the floor scrupulously clean.
- Keep a box for tidying away toys and clutter.

WASTEBINS
- Discourage toddlers from rummaging in the wastebin.
- Put sharp-edged cans and lids or broken glass straight into the dustbin.
- Keep the wastebin in a cupboard with a child-resistant safety catch.

> **KEEP** *a fire blanket in the kitchen for smothering flare-ups. If you want to buy a fire extinguisher, consult your local fire brigade to find out which is the most appropriate type. For more on fires, see p.11 and p.112.*

Babies

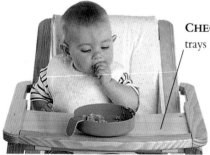

CHECK that removable trays have strong clasps

ATTACH a safety harness to the clips on either side of the chair

BOTTLES AND FOOD
- Sterilise all your baby's feeding equipment.
- Don't leave a prepared feed standing at room temperature, and don't keep the remains of the last feed. Warmed or reheated feeds are breeding grounds for bacteria that might upset your baby's stomach.

HIGHCHAIRS
- Always use a safety harness.
- Never leave the chair where your baby can reach out and pull objects down from a surface. Keep him amused with a safe toy.
- Never leave your child unattended.

PLAY
- Have a safe area or a playpen where your baby can play and watch you.
- Keep him out of range of any spills from the cooker.

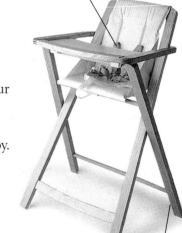

CHOOSE a stable highchair with widely spaced legs.

TABLES AND WORK SURFACES

- Always be aware of your child's reach and keep all heavy, breakable, or sharp objects well back from the edges of surfaces.
- Keep stools or chairs away from tables and work surfaces to prevent your child from climbing up on them.
- Tuck flexes of kettles, toasters, blenders, and irons out of reach. Choose a curly flex for your kettle if possible. It is not only boiling, steaming kettles that pose a hazard: water is still hot enough to scald 15 minutes after boiling.
- Leave electrical appliances unplugged when they are not in use.
- Avoid using a tablecloth. It is tempting for a crawling baby or toddler to use it to pull himself up, bringing anything on the table down upon his head. Use table mats instead, or secure the cloth with clips.
- Do not put your baby on a table or work surface when he is in a car seat or bouncing cradle: he could easily fall off.

CUPBOARDS AND DRAWERS

- Put safety catches on cupboards and drawers, particularly those that contain: knives, scissors, and cutlery; heavy pots, pans, or china; dried food, such as lentils or pasta, that may be a choking hazard; alcohol and bottles; medicines, including vitamins; cleaning materials, such as washing powder or bleach, including those with "child-resistant" lids.

FRIDGE

Food poisoning can be caused by poor food storage. Take precautions to minimise risks:
- Keep cooked meat and poultry on a separate shelf from uncooked meat. Cover uncooked meat with kitchen film.
- Don't store food in open tins; tip leftovers into a clean container and put in the fridge.
- Check food regularly, to see that nothing is kept beyond the "sell-by" date.

COOKER

Your child is obviously at risk of burns and scalds from hot fat or boiling water when you are preparing food.
- You can buy safety guards, but remember that a child can still poke fingers through some types and be burnt by hot hobs or gas rings.
- Always keep your child away from oven doors; they can get very hot while the oven is in use and will stay hot for some time afterwards. A crawling baby or toddler is particularly at risk. Try to teach your child what "hot" means so that he understands a warning.
- Keep matches well out of reach in a cupboard with a safety catch.

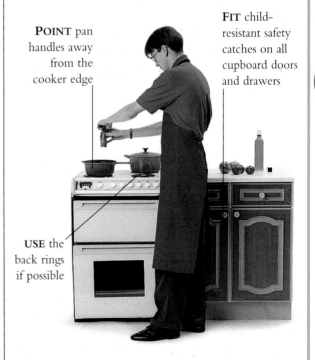

POINT pan handles away from the cooker edge

FIT child-resistant safety catches on all cupboard doors and drawers

USE the back rings if possible

WASHING MACHINE AND TUMBLE DRIER

- Keep small hands away from the glass door; it may get hot while the machine is on.
- Ensure the door is closed while the machine is not in use. Your toddler may try to climb inside or fill it with toys.

SITTING ROOM

While your children are very young, try to arrange the room so that both children and your valuables are kept out of harm's way. If you have a balcony, block up gaps in the railings with hardboard and check that your child can't climb over. Never leave toys on a high surface as he may attempt to retrieve them.

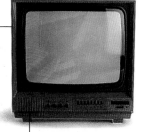

CARPETS AND CURTAINS

- Check that there are no areas of carpet or rug that have holes or turned up edges; either you or your child could trip up.
- Wind up and tuck away curtain ties and cords for blinds. Children can be strangled if they get caught in dangling cords.

FIREPLACES AND HEATERS

- Don't leave matches or cigarette lighters where your child can reach them.
- Use a fireguard over an open fire. Fix it to the wall to prevent your child pulling it over. Put a guard over gas heaters.
- Never use the fireguard as a shelf or clothes airer.
- Use a spark-guard as well as a fireguard for open fires as an additional precaution.

TELEVISIONS, VIDEOS, AND HI-FI EQUIPMENT

- Fix wiring to the skirting board.
- Run long flexes behind furniture so that your child won't trip or pull on them.

POSITION electrical equipment against the wall so that your child can't get at the back

- Cover unused plug sockets with safety covers.
- Check that old flexes are not worn.
- Ensure that the TV cannot be pulled over.

SURFACES AND FURNITURE

- Place house plants out of reach of young children. Some house plants are poisonous, and others can scratch or produce allergic reactions if touched.
- Keep breakable or heavy objects off low tables and well back from the edges of surfaces such as window sills or mantelpieces.
- Remove glass-topped tables and put corner protectors on sharp table corners.
- Don't leave hot drinks, alcohol, glasses, cigarettes, matches, or lighters on low surfaces, such as coffee tables, where your child can reach them.
  - Keep alcohol in a locked cupboard.
  - Never leave a cigarette burning on the arm of a sofa or armchair. Old foam furniture can be lethal in a fire as it releases toxic fumes within seconds of catching alight.

116

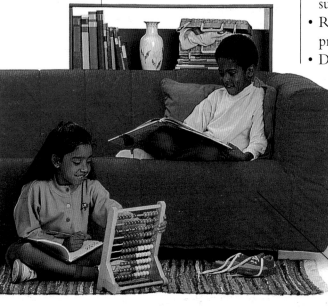

ENSURE bookcases are secured to the wall

ENSURE sofas and armchairs have fire-resistant fillings and coverings

TOYS AND PLAYTHINGS

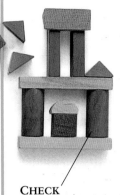

When you buy toys or equipment for your child, follow these guidelines:

- Buy toys that are appropriate for the age of your child, and buy from a reputable source.
- Make sure that there are no sharp edges, and avoid anything made of thin, rigid plastic.
- Buy non-toxic paints or crayons.
- Don't buy your child second-hand toys: they may be covered in paint containing lead.
- Avoid novelty toys that are not designed to be played with by young children: look out for warnings on the packaging.

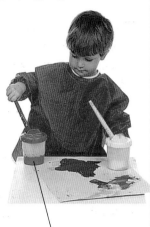

CHECK that sets of building blocks don't have small pieces that could be a choking hazard for your child

GIVE your child non-toxic paints to play with

CARING FOR TOYS

- Check toys regularly and throw away any broken ones.
- Don't mix batteries – change them all at the same time, otherwise the strong batteries will make the weak ones very hot.
- Keep toys in a toy box. Toys can bring about accidents or injuries by being left on the floor.

117

Babies and toddlers

- Remove ribbons from a baby's soft toys.
- Check that the eyes, noses, ears, or bells on soft toys and dolls are well secured.
- Attach cot toys with a very short string and remove them as soon as your baby can sit up.
- Remove activity centres or bulky toys from a cot as soon as your child can stand because they provide a foothold for climbing out.
- Don't let babies chew on furry toys: the fur is a choking hazard.
- Never let a young child play with a toy that is not recommended for his age-group: it may contain small pieces on which he could choke.
- Always supervise a baby or toddler while he is playing.
- Do not use baby walkers.

MAKE SURE that toys that increase mobility are stable

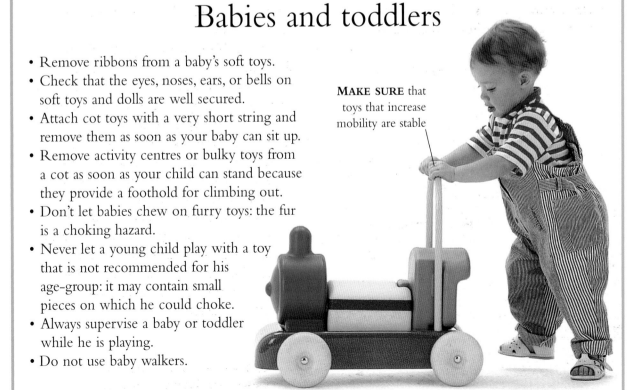

BEDROOMS

The cupboards and drawers in bedrooms are always exciting places for toddlers and young children. Make sure any potentially hazardous items are out of reach, as you may not always know when your child will decide to go exploring on his own.

Babies

COT

- Make sure the cot is deep enough to prevent your baby from climbing out – at least 50cm (1ft 8in) from the top of the mattress to the top of the cot.
- Bar spaces must be between 2.5 and 6cm (1–2⅜in) wide to prevent your baby's head from being trapped.

- The mattress must be the right size with a gap no larger than 3cm (1⅛in) around the side. Otherwise, the baby's head could get trapped between the side of the cot and the mattress.
- Do not use a pillow for a baby under one year: it could suffocate him. If you need to raise his head, put a pillow underneath the mattress.
- Use a sheet and cellular blankets rather than a duvet until your baby is a year old. Your baby could overheat or suffocate under a duvet.
- Always put your baby to sleep on his back with his feet at the foot of the cot to lessen the risk of cot death.
- Remove bumpers as soon as your baby can sit up because he could use them to climb out.
- Once he starts trying to climb out of the cot, transfer him to a bed. You can fit a bed guard at first, until he is used to the bed.

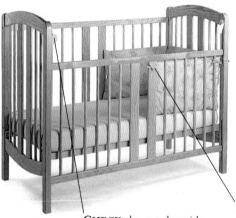

CHECK the cot dropside has strong clasps that your baby cannot open

ENSURE that bumpers have very short ties to prevent strangulation

CHANGING AREA

- Keep all changing equipment in one area so that you never have to leave your baby alone. He will be safest on the floor, but if you have a changing table, remember that he might roll off if left for even a moment.
- Do not have shelves above the changing area in case something falls off.
- Keep mobiles out of his reach.
- If you use talcum powder, sprinkle it on your hands and rub them together to avoid creating a cloud of dust around your baby.

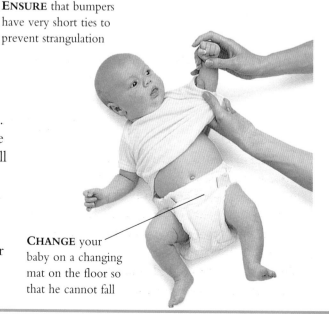

CHANGE your baby on a changing mat on the floor so that he cannot fall

Your child's room

BEDS
- Use a bed guard when your toddler first moves to a bed.
- Top bunk beds must have safety rails on both sides and any gaps in the railings or between the top of the mattress and the bottom of the safety rail should be no more than 6–7.5cm (2½–3in).
- A top bunk is not recommended for children under the age of six.
- Never let young children play on the top bunk.
- Remove toys from the floor by the bed at night.

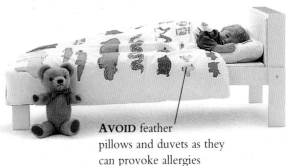

AVOID feather pillows and duvets as they can provoke allergies

WINDOWS
Make sure your child can't climb out. Even if his room is on the ground floor, he is in danger if he falls.
- Fix a safety catch, but make sure the window can be opened easily in the event of a fire.
- Try not to place a piece of furniture below a window because it may encourage your child to climb up.

TOYS (see p. 117).
- Try to keep toys with small pieces separate from others so that you can easily remove them and put them out of reach for a while if your child is sharing a room with a toddler, or if you have young visitors.

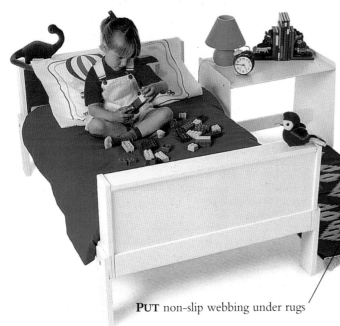

PUT non-slip webbing under rugs

119

Your room

- **Medicines and pills** Do not keep them beside your bed or on a dressing table. Put them out of sight and out of reach.
- **Scissors and sewing equipment** Keep these in a drawer or cupboard where your child cannot reach them.
- **Perfume, hairspray, and makeup** These can be harmful if sprayed or rubbed in the eyes,

or drunk, so keep them out of reach or in a drawer with a safety catch.
- **China cups and glasses** Never leave a china cup or a glass on the floor by your bed. If your child is sleeping in your bed at night and rolls out onto the cup or the glass, he could have a serious accident.

BATHROOM

Your child may be at risk from falls, drowning, or poisoning in the bathroom. Keep the bathroom door shut at all times to discourage him from going in. On the inside of the door, fix the bolt high up to prevent a small child locking himself in.

SHOWER
- Keep a constant check on the temperature of the water.
- Use non-slip mats in the shower and on the bathroom floor.
- Put safety film on a glass shower door so that glass is held in place in case of an accident.

BATH
- Always check the temperature of the water before your child gets in. A young child can be badly scalded by hot bath water.
- Use non-slip mats in the bath and on the floor by the bath.
- Never leave a young child or baby alone in the bath. A baby can drown in just 2.5cm (1in) of water. If you need to answer the doorbell or telephone, take your child with you.

CUPBOARDS AND CABINETS
- Store bathroom chemicals and other potential poisons, such as toilet cleaners and bleach, out of reach in a cupboard with a safety catch.
- Keep other hazards, such as make-up, aftershave, razors, nail scissors, and any medicines or glass containers, out of reach in a locked medicine cabinet.

TOILET
- Use a special child toilet seat adaptor and step for toddlers so that they can keep their balance more easily and so feel more secure.
- Keep the toilet seat closed.
- Don't use block toilet cleaners that a small child could pull out and chew.
- Never mix toilet cleaners with bleach as this can give off toxic fumes.
- If your toddler uses a potty, keep it clean, but never leave bleach or cleaning agents inside it.

120

BATH him away from the tap end

NEVER leave your child unattended in the bath

USE a non-slip mat in the bath

GARDEN

Your garden can be a safe and interesting place for your children to play. Children will find their own corners to play in but you should remove obvious hazards:

- Clear away any rubbish or rubble.
- Check garden furniture or play equipment regularly to make sure that it is stable, safe, and sited over a soft surface, such as grass.
- Keep pets off areas where children play.
- Make sure paving is even and remove moss: children may easily trip or slip.
- Lock gates that lead out of the garden and make sure fences are secure.

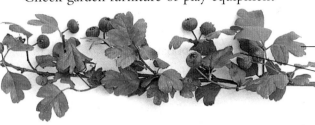

WARN your child not to eat berries or leaves

PLANTS

Many plants are poisonous if eaten and digested in large quantities. Small pieces, or one or two berries, are not fatal but may cause some discomfort and stomach upset.

- Tell your child about the dangers of eating berries, and keep babies and toddlers away from them.
- Remove plants that you know to be poisonous, such as deadly nightshade, laburnum, and toadstools.
- Cut back any prickly plants, such as roses, brambles, and holly – they can give nasty scratches, especially to the eyes.

SUPERVISE your toddler at all times. Check that he is playing in a clean, safe area with safe toys

SHEDS

These are exciting dens for children.

- If your shed is full of gardening equipment or tools, tell your child that it is out of bounds and keep it locked.
- Put any chemicals, such as weedkiller or slug pellets, out of reach.

PONDS, PADDLING POOLS, AND WATER BUTTS

Children are in danger if they slip and fall, even in shallow water.

- Never leave children unattended when they are playing in, or near, water.
- Cover ponds, water butts, and empty dustbins that collect rainwater.
- Always empty out a paddling pool when your children have finished playing in it and turn it upside-down in case it rains.

GARDENING

- Don't put down chemicals when children will be playing in the garden.
- Don't mow the lawn while children are close by because stone chips may become dislodged and fly up into their eyes.
- Put away all garden tools when you have finished using them.

121

OUT AND ABOUT

After the home, most accidents to children occur in the street. Teach your child the rules of the road from an early age, reminding him to stay alert for traffic and to cross in a safe place. It takes a long time for children to develop a true road sense.

AS A GENERAL GUIDE:
- Three-year-olds can learn that the pavement is safe and the road is dangerous.
- Five-year-olds can learn how to cross the road, but they are still not able to put this knowledge into practice on their own.
- Eight-year-olds can cross quiet streets on their own, but are not yet able to judge the speed and distance of traffic.
- Twelve-year-olds can judge the speed of an oncoming car, but are still easily distracted by friends.

IN THE STREET
Whenever you are out with your child, show him how to be aware of his own safety.
- Use reins or a wrist strap for a toddler, to stop him running off.
- Hold a young child's hand when you are near the road or waiting to cross.
- Teach your child by example and always find a safe place to cross. This may be:

  ▲ *A zebra crossing – wait at the island halfway, if there is one.*

  ▲ *A pelican crossing at traffic lights. Encourage your child to press the button and tell him to wait until the traffic has stopped.*

  ▲ *An underpass.*

  ▲ *A footbridge.*

  ▲ *A large gap between parked cars, where your child can see a long way in both directions.*

Crossing the road
Teach your child the rules of the road:

▲ *Find a safe place to cross, then stop.*

▲ *Stand on the pavement, near the kerb.*

▲ *Look all around for traffic, and listen.*

▲ *If traffic is coming, let it pass.*

▲ *When there is no traffic near, walk straight across the road.*

▲ *Keep looking and listening for traffic while you cross.*

BIKES
- Children under 10 years old should not cycle on roads in traffic without adult supervision.
- Arrange for your child to have cycle training before he starts on the roads.
- Make sure your child can be seen when he's riding his bike – with bright fluorescent colours by day and reflectors on his clothes and bike by night. He should wear an approved helmet to protect his head.

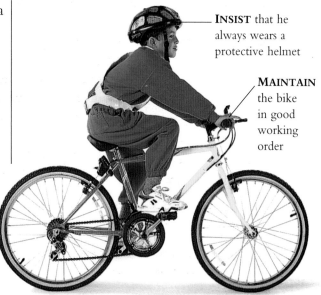

INSIST that he always wears a protective helmet

MAINTAIN the bike in good working order

PLAYING

What may seem common sense to you is not always obvious to children.

- Teach your child the dangers of playing in open areas, such as roads, building sites, and quarries.
- Tell your child not to play in the street, or on a pavement near the kerb.
- Tell him that he must never chase a ball, a pet, or another child into the road.
- Tell him not to try to cross the road from between two closely parked cars.

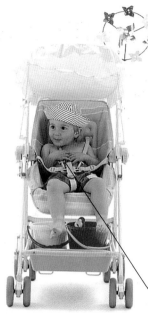

PRAMS AND BUGGIES

- Never push a pram or buggy out into the traffic – pull it to one side and check whether it is safe to cross. Remember that a buggy sticks out in front of you by at least 1m (3ft).
- When you park a pram or buggy, put on the brakes and point it away from traffic.
- Never tie your dog to the pram.
- Never leave a baby unattended.

HARNESS your baby into his buggy

In the playground

Playgrounds should comply with safety standards and recommendations.

- The play area must be safely fenced off and away from roads.
- There should be a soft, even surface, such as bark chippings or rubber tiles, around equipment.
- Slides should be no higher than 2.4m (8ft) and preferably constructed on an earth mound to break any falls.
- Roundabouts should be low, with a smooth surface, designed so that children can't get their feet stuck underneath.
- Climbing frames should be no higher than 2.4m (8ft), completely stable, and built over sand or a very soft surface to break falls.
  - There should be a clearly defined play area for toddlers and young children, set away from the more boisterous activities of older children.
  - There should be someone to contact if equipment is faulty.
  - Dogs must not be allowed inside playgrounds.

CHECK that swings are set apart from main play equipment, or fenced off, to prevent children running in front of, or behind, them

MAKE SURE your child is wearing suitable clothing

TEACH your child how to use equipment properly

STRANGERS *Remind your child of the dangers of talking to strangers. Have a code word that a friend can use if meeting your child. Tell your child not to go with anybody unless they use the code.*

GARAGE & CAR SAFETY

GARAGE

- Keep the garage locked and discourage your child from going in there.
- Keep equipment, chemicals, or tools out of your child's reach and locked away if possible.
- Make sure you know where your child is when you are driving into, or out of, the garage.
- If you keep a freezer in the garage, it should be locked at all times.

CAR

- Never leave a young child unattended in a car.
- Don't let your child play with the windows, whether manual or electric. Windows can trap a child's head or fingers.
- Remove the cigarette lighter.
- Watch out for your child's fingers when you shut the doors.
- Use child locks on rear doors until your child is at least six years old.
- Teach your child to get out of the car on the pavement side.
- If your child is helping you as you wash or tidy the car, make sure you have removed the keys from the ignition.

CAR SEATS

Always put your child into a special safety seat when you strap him into the car. Do not buy a second-hand car seat because some car seats are reconditioned after a crash and will not be safe. Choose the right seat for the weight and development of your child:

- **Babies** up to 13kg (29lb) – about nine months – should travel in a rear-facing car seat. The baby is harnessed into the seat and the seat is held in place by the car seat belts. The safest place for your baby to travel is on the rear seat of your car. Make sure you do not place your baby in a rear-facing car seat on the front passenger seat if there is an airbag fitted because the impact of an airbag inflating could cause him serious head or neck injuries.
- Never carry a baby on your lap or inside your own seatbelt: he would be crushed in a crash.
- **Older babies and toddlers**, up to 18kg (40lb), need a car seat in the back of the car. Some of these seats have an integral harness for the child, which fits over his shoulders and between his legs. These seats are kept in place by the adult seat belt, or by straps that you can fix into the car. Other types of seat use the adult belt to hold both the child and the seat in the car.
- **Primary school children** should travel in a booster seat. Without it, adult seat belts are neither comfortable nor safe: the shoulder part cuts across the child's neck, and the lap strap lies across his stomach. In a crash, the lap strap can damage a child's liver or spleen. A booster seat raises a young child so that the shoulder part lies across his upper chest and the lap strap lies across his hips. A lap strap on its own is not sufficient as it does not restrain the child's upper body.

FIT a child car seat for maximum protection

24

INDEX

126

127

Acknowledgments

PREVIOUS EDITION
Project Editor Caroline Greene **Senior Art Editor** Jane Bull **Managing Editor** Jemima Dunne **Managing Art Editor** Tina Vaughan **DTP Designer** Karen Ruane **Production** Maryann Rogers **Photography** Andy Crawford, Steve Gorton

Dorling Kindersley would like to thank:
Charlotte Stark and Dr Mike Hayes of the Child Accident Prevention Trust for reviewing *Safety In and Around the Home*; Hilary Bird for the index; the following for modelling:
Children Aleena Awan, Navaz Awan, Amy Davies, Thomas Davies, James Dow, Kyla Edwards, Austin Enil, Lia Foa, Maya Foa, Kashi Gorton, Emily Gorton, Thomas Greene, Alexander Harrison, Rupert Harrison, Ben Harrison, Jessica Harris-Voss, Jake Hutton, Rosemary Kaloki, Winnie Kaloki, Ella Kaye, Maddy Kaye, Jade Lamb, Emily Leney, Crispin Lord, Daniel Lord, Harriet Lord, Ailsa McCaughrean, Fiona Maine, Tom Maine, Maija Marsh, Oliver Metcalf, Eloise Morgan, Tom Razazan, Jimmy Razazan, Georgia Ritter, Rebecca Sharples, Ben Sharples, Thomas Sharples, Ben Walker, Robyn Walker, Amy Beth Walton Evans, Hanna Warren-Green, Simon Weekes, Joseph Weir, Lily Ziegler
Adults Shaila Awan, Claire le Bas, Joanna Benwell, Georgina Davies, Marion Davies, Sophie Dow, Jemima Dunne, Tina Edwards, Rachel Fitchett, Emma Foa, Caroline Greene, Susan Harrison, Victoria Harrison, Julia Harris-Voss, Emma Hutton, Helga Lien Evans, Sylvie Jordan, Jane Kaloki, David Kaye, Louise Kaye, Philip Lord, Geraldine McCaughrean, Diana Maine, Brian Marsh, Jonathan Metcalf, Francoise Morgan, Hossein Razazan, Angela Sharples, John Sharples, Miranda Tunbridge, Vanessa Walker, Catherine Warren-Green, Toni Weekes, Robert Ziegler

Make-up: Wendy Holmes, Pebbles, Geoff Portas
Additional photographs Dave King, Ray Mollers, Suzannah Price, Dave Rudkin, Steve Shott

EMERGENCY TELEPHONE NUMBERS

> **IN AN EMERGENCY GO TO THE NEAREST TELEPHONE AND DIAL 999. ASK FOR THE POLICE, AMBULANCE OR FIRE BRIGADE**

DOCTOR
Name: _____
Address: _____
_____
Telephone: _____
Surgery Hours: _____

HEALTH VISITOR
Name: _____
Clinic Address: _____
_____
Telephone: _____
Clinic Hours: _____

DENTIST
Name: _____
Address: _____
_____
Telephone: _____
Surgery Hours: _____

HOSPITAL ACCIDENT & EMERGENCY
Address: _____
_____
Telephone: _____

LATE NIGHT CHEMIST
Address: _____
_____

LOCAL POLICE STATION
Address: _____
_____
Telephone: _____

GAS EMERGENCY SERVICE
Telephone: _____

ELECTRICITY EMERGENCY SERVICE
Telephone: _____

WATER EMERGENCY SERVICE
Telephone: _____

TAXI
Telephone: _____

IN CASE OF AN EMERGENCY PLEASE CALL: _____
_____

British Red Cross

The British Red Cross runs first aid courses for all ages.
For further information, get in touch with your local British Red Cross office; you will find the number in the telephone directory or in the Yellow Pages. Alternatively, visit www.redcross.org.uk.

British Red Cross
UK Office
9 Grosvenor Crescent
London SW1X 7EJ
020 7235 5454

The Red Cross emblem is a symbol of protection during armed conflicts, and its use is restricted by law.

Details of the royalties payable to the British Red Cross can be obtained by writing to the publisher Dorling Kindersley at the following address: 80 Strand, London, WC2R 0RL

128